EASY BREAD MAKING
FOR SPECIAL DIETS

Wheat-free, Milk- and Lactose-free,
Egg-free, Gluten-free, Yeast-free, Sugar-free,
Low Fat, High or Low Fiber, Low Sodium,
Diabetic, and Low Calorie

Use your bread machine,
food processor, or mixer to make the bread
YOU need quickly and easily

By
Nicolette M. Dumke

EASY BREADMAKING FOR SPECIAL DIETS: USE YOUR BREAD MACHINE, FOOD PROCESSOR, OR MIXER TO MAKE THE BREAD YOU NEED QUICKLY AND EASILY

Published by
Adapt Books
Allergy Adapt, Inc.
1877 Polk Avenue
Louisville, Colorado 80027
(303) 666-8253

©1995 by Nicolette M. Dumke
Fourth Printing, April, 1999
Printed in the United States of America

Cover design and typography by Ed Nies, Mel Typesetting,
1519 S. Pearl St., Denver, Colorado 80210, (303) 777-5571

10   9   8   7   6   5   4

Publisher's Cataloging in Publication Data

Dumke, Nicolette M.
    Easy Breadmaking for Special Diets: use your bread machine, food processor, or mixer to make the bread YOU need quickly and easily / Nicolette M. Dumke.
256 p.   4 cm.
Includes bibliographical references and index.
ISBN: 1-887624-02-3

1. Bread.   2. Diet therapy.   I. Title

TX769.D86 1996   641.8'15
                                                 QBI95-20288
Library of Congress Catalog Card Number: 95-77917
$14.95

Dedication

To my husband Mark,
for his encouragement and support of all of my efforts,

To my son Joel,
for his optimism and positive attitude,

To my son John,
my best helper with this book, who with his adventuresome
spirit tasted every loaf,

And to my many other tasters:
my mother, Mary Jiannetti,
my sister, Gina Jiannetti,
and numerous friends.

DISCLAIMER

The information contained in this book is merely intended to communicate food preparation material which is helpful and educational to the reader. It is not intended to replace medical diagnosis or treatment, but rather to provide recipes which may be helpful in implementing a diet prescribed by your doctor. Please consult your physician for medical advice before changing your diet.

The author and publisher declare that to the best of their knowledge all material in this book is accurate; however, although unknown to the author and publisher, some recipes may contain ingredients which may be harmful to some people.

There are no warranties which extend beyond the educational nature of this book. Therefore, we shall have neither liability nor responsibility to any person with respect to any loss or damage alleged to be caused, directly or indirectly, by the information contained in this book.

Table of Contents

Foreword

Like the indescribable aroma of fresh baked bread, wafting from the kitchens of our childhood, comes this wonderful book all about bread.

Easy Breadmaking for Special Diets considers making dozens of different kinds of bread from a wide variety of flours, some of whose names you may have never even heard. It deals with making bread by many techniques, from "by hand" to using the most sophisticated equipment and ovens available. It analyzes the nutritional values of the recipes for you, and shows you how to fit bread into any health-conscious diet.

It offers hope to the environmentally sensitive person who has become resigned to giving up the comfort of having bread as a basic part of any meal. The author shows you how to make really good bread without yeast, milk, eggs, wheat, or salt — all those things you thought were absolutely essential for bread making.

This is a book for people who want to make more bread, for people who want to start making bread, and for people, who because of their allergies, are afraid to make bread. It's all here for you. Enjoy!

Elizabeth Pinar, M.S., R.D.

Medical Nutrition Consultant in
    private practice

Dietetics Educator – Master Teacher
    Emeritus, Front Range
    Community College

Author of menu planning software,
    including *Dinner! for Windows*

Bread, the Staff of Life

Bread is the most basic of all foods; it is called the staff of life. Without it, our diets do not seem complete. For 2000 years, people have been asking, "Give us this day our daily bread." The USDA's new food guide pyramid tells us that breads and grains should be the largest part of a health-promoting diet. And yet, those of us on special diets may find it difficult or impossible to purchase commercially made bread that conforms to the diets we must follow for good health.

But there is no reason to despair. We can make our own bread quickly and easily. We can take charge of our health and take charge of our life. We can be in control of what we eat, and will find that our homemade bread tastes better than anything we have eaten before. Our homes smell wonderful when we bake. If we want to have bread that will keep us healthy on our special diets, we can make our own.

When you first embark upon a special diet, the challenge of making all of your own bread can seem overwhelming, but with the many labor-saving devices now available, it does not have to be difficult or take all day like it used to for our grandmothers. Mixers and food processors can do the heavy work of kneading dough, microwave ovens can help it rise in record time, or a bread machine can do the whole job for you from start to finish.

The purpose of this book is to help you achieve good health by following your special diet and to enjoy the simple pleasures of homemade bread while saving you time and effort in the kitchen. The investment you make in good health for yourself and those you love is well worth the effort involved.

Special Diets, Special Recipes

Special diets are used to treat and control a wide variety of medical conditions. Even your family members who consider themselves normal and healthy can benefit from taking control of what goes into their mouths and what goes into their bread. We are what we eat!

Food allergies are commonly treated by avoiding the foods that you are allergic to, such as wheat, milk, eggs, and yeast. Many people cannot handle lactose because they lack the enzyme needed to digest it and so must avoid milk. Individuals with celiac disease must avoid all gluten. People with heart disease or high blood pressure must limit the amount of sodium and/or fat and cholesterol they eat. Diabetics must strictly control the amount of all nutrients and calories they consume, balancing their food intake against their insulin intake or production. People with intestinal diseases may need either high fiber or low fiber diets. And all of us are told that low fat, high fiber diets are good for the prevention of many diseases, such as cancer and heart disease. In this chapter, we will consider some special diets and the recipes in this book that you can use when you are on them.

WHEAT-FREE DIETS

At first glance, a wheat-free diet presents a great challenge to a person baking bread. Wheat is the basic ingredient of almost all commercial bread. Before 1990, those of us with wheat allergies were resigned to eating very dense bread, but with the introduction of spelt to the American market, we once again can make light, fluffy, yet wheat-free breads.

Spelt is a grain that is closely related to wheat. Many individuals who are allergic to wheat can tolerate spelt, but be sure to consult your doctor before trying it. If you can eat spelt, you can have almost any kind of bread you want, and your friends and family may never know it does not contain wheat. Spelt flour is the basis for many of the wheat-free breads in this book.

For those who "rotate" their grains as part of an allergy diet, this book contains recipes for breads made with single grains besides spelt, such as barley, rye, oats, kamut, and rice, and the non-grains, buckwheat, amaranth, and quinoa. (See page 84 and pages 88 to 98.) Using these recipes, you can eat bread made with a different grain or non-grain on each day of your rotation diet. If you must also rotate or avoid yeast, refer to pages 145 and 147-152 for yeast-free, single grain recipes.

Over half of the recipes in this book are wheat-free. If you are on a wheat-free diet, avoid those recipes that contain bread flour, all purpose flour, whole wheat flour, whole wheat bread flour, gluten flour, or wheat germ. Also, see the index of wheat-free recipes beginning on page 239.

GLUTEN-FREE DIETS

People with celiac disease (gluten sensitive enteropathy) must avoid all gluten in their diets. Although independent testing laboratories, such as the Rodale Institute, find grains such as millet, milo, and teff and the non-grains amaranth, quinoa, and buckwheat to be essentially gluten-free, the Celiac Sprue Association has not yet tested these flours and recommends eating breads made from only rice, potato, tapioca, arrowroot, corn, and legume flours. For gluten-free recipes, refer to the listing of rice recipes on page 240.

MILK- AND LACTOSE-FREE DIETS

It may be necessary to avoid milk products in the diet for several reasons. Some individuals lack the enzyme lactase that breaks lactose (milk sugar) down into glucose and galactose. When the undigested lactose enters the intestine, it causes cramping, gas, and diarrhea. Some lactase-deficient people can tolerate small amounts of milk products, such as the amounts usually found in commercial breads, or can use lactase-treated milk in their diets.

Others must avoid milk in their diets because of allergy to the protein components of milk. These people must usually strictly avoid all milk in their foods. If tolerated, soy or rice milk may be used as a milk substitute in cooking, but it usually works just as well to substitute water. With the exception of "Calzones," p. 185 to 186, "Mexican Strata," p. 187, and "Pizza," p. 180 to 183, where cheese is an optional ingredient, all of the recipes in this book are milk- and lactose-free and are suitable for those on milk- and lactose-free diets.

EGG-FREE DIETS

Your doctor may recommend an egg-free diet for a variety of reasons. The most common reason today is to control cholesterol levels for the prevention or treatment of heart disease. Most of the recipes in this book are egg-free. A few of the gluten-free recipes require eggs to give structure to the bread, but if you are avoiding eggs to control your cholesterol, a cholesterol-free egg substitute may be used in place of the eggs in these recipes, and is given as an alternative ingredient.

Those who must avoid eggs in their diet because of food allergies should also avoid egg substitutes because they contain egg white, which for most people is the most allergenic part of the egg. Only the cholesterol-rich yolk has been removed in commercial egg substitutes. Egg substitutes may also contain milk or milk derivatives, corn derivatives, or even wheat gluten, all of which can be very allergenic. If you are allergic to both gluten-containing grains and eggs, you may have to settle for dense bread, but such bread is still much better than no bread at all.

SUGAR-FREE DIETS

At our house we have a saying, "Sugar isn't good for anybody." In our experience, we have found that eliminating sugar from our diets is the best way to control our weight without feeling hungry, counting calories, limiting portion sizes, or making any other changes. On a sugar-free diet, wide swings in blood sugar levels, which can lead to excessive hunger and overeating, are uncommon. Eating a large amount of sugar may also predispose to the development of dental cavities, candidiasis, heart disease (by raising the level of blood fats), adult onset diabetes (by "wearing out" the pancreas), and a number of other diseases.

Sugar can be replaced in your diet with fruit and fruit sweeteners. Once your taste buds have become used to a sugar-free diet, treats made with fruit sweeteners are just as delicious and satisfying as those made with sugar. All of the recipes in this book are sugar-free except for the optional sweet roll and doughnut glazes. Honey is given as an optional alternative ingredient to fruit sweeteners in a few of the sweet bread and roll recipes for those whose taste buds may desire a little more intensely sweet taste than the fruit sweeteners contribute. Molasses is used in the Pumpernickel Bread, Brown Bread, and Gingerbread recipes.

YEAST-FREE DIETS

Yeast is a common food allergen, and must be avoided by many people with food allergies. However, it is possible to make very enjoyable yeast-free breads. There are several bread machines on the market that have a cake or quick bread cycle that can make yeast-free breads. Making yeast-free breads by hand is also very easy. For yeast-free bread recipes, see pages 52 to 54 and pages 144 to 162. Also, be sure to read "All About Quick Breads" on pages 16 to 17.

HEART HEALTHY, LOW FAT, AND LOW CHOLESTEROL DIETS

People on heart healthy diets are usually advised to control the amount of saturated fat and cholesterol they consume. All of the recipes in this book are made with minimal amounts of oil rather than saturated fats such as butter or margarine. Some types of oil, such as canola or olive oil, may be considered better for the prevention or treatment of heart disease than other kinds of oils. Ask your doctor or nutritionist what type of oil you should use.

As mentioned above in the section on egg-free diets, except when necessary to add structure to gluten-free breads, all of the recipes in this book are egg-free. If you are not allergic to eggs or the other ingredients in commercial egg substitutes and wish to make gluten-free breads, you may want to use an egg substitute to avoid the cholesterol in eggs. A few recipes in this book, most of them in the main dish section, pages 175 to 189, contain a small amount of cholesterol, but most of the recipes in this book are free of all saturated fat and cholesterol. Refer to the nutritional analyses of specific recipes to see if the saturated fat and cholesterol level in them is low enough to conform to the diet your doctor has given you.

LOW SODIUM DIETS

A low sodium, or low salt, diet may be recommended for the treatment of high blood pressure, heart disease, or kidney disease. Most of the sodium in our diets comes from salt added to foods. Low sodium bread is a special challenge because salt moderates and controls the growth of the yeast in bread, and also contributes to the strength of the gluten structure. Therefore, omitting salt in a bread that has a less-than-perfect gluten structure to begin with will cause the bread to fall. A few recipes are included in this book that contain no added salt. (See pages 62, 64, and 70.) If you are on a sodium restricted diet and wish to make the other recipes using less salt, the amount of salt in the recipe may be cut in half, which will almost cut the sodium content of the bread in half, without affecting the quality of the bread too much, although the taste will be different. Or consider eliminating the salt from what you put on the bread (butter, nut butter, meat, etc.) rather than from the bread itself.

HIGH FIBER DIETS

High fiber diets are recommended for the treatment of constipation, diverticulosis, irritable bowel syndrome, and hemorrhoids. A high fiber diet may also help stabilize blood sugar levels for diabetics and hypoglycemics by slowing down and stabilizing the rate at which glucose is absorbed from the digestive system. High fiber diets also help control blood cholesterol levels and may help prevent cancer and heart disease. The USDA's new food pyramid and food guidelines recommend generous amounts of fiber for almost everyone.

There are two types of fiber, soluble and insoluble. Insoluble fiber, such as is present in wheat bran and rice bran, passes through the digestive system unchanged and prevents constipation. Soluble fiber, such as is present in apples, barley, and oats, is broken down by the bacteria in the large intestine. It is useful for the prevention of cancer and heart disease.

Grains in general and many of the breads in this book are good sources of fiber. For high fiber bread recipes, refer to pages 69 to 73 and "Whole Grain and Extra-Nutrition Breads," pages 79 to 109.

LOW FIBER DIETS

People who have inflammatory bowel diseases may need to eat low fiber diets to keep from further irritating their intestine. I "discovered" white spelt flour while trying to find low fiber wheat alternatives for a friend who has ulcerative colitis. While insoluble fiber can be a problem for those with IBD, soluble fiber can be a friend. Oatmeal is often recommended as a home remedy for flareups because it contains a lot of soluble fiber which absorbs water and slows transit time through the intestine. Because I am allergic to grains, I have not tried the "oatmeal remedy," but have found other soluble fibers, such as psyllium seed, guar gum, and apple pectin, helpful for Crohn's disease.

Many of the basic bread recipes in this book are low enough in fiber for a low fiber diet. Refer to the nutritional analyses of the recipes to get an idea of how much fiber each recipe contains and how likely you are to tolerate it. Much of the fiber in the Oatmeal Breads, pages 72 to 73, is soluble fiber, so oatmeal bread may be tolerated better than the oat bran breads or other whole grain breads which are high in insoluble fiber. Also, there are rice bread recipes made with white rice flour rather than brown rice flour (see pages 50, 54, 76, and 152) and white rye flour recipes (see pages 89, 90 and 149) that may be useful for those on low fiber diets.

DIABETIC DIETS

Diabetics must strictly control their intake of calories and nutrients, and balance their food consumption against their insulin intake or their body's production of insulin. This is usually accomplished by using a system of "exchanges" to budget and control their intake of various nutrients.

Your doctor or dietician will work out a diet for you which tells you how many of which food exchanges to eat at each meal and snack. The serving sizes for the recipes in this book have been geared to the diabetic exchange system. For example, the nutritional analysis for a dense, whole grain bread may say that a large loaf of bread contains 22 servings. Each serving will contain about 80 calories and 15 grams of carbohydrate and be one starch/bread exchange. However, when you make the bread in a bread machine, you may get a 6 inch tall loaf, which is difficult to cut into 22 slices. A diabetic can cut the loaf into 11 horizontal slices and count each half slice as one starch/bread exchange. A person who is not a diabetic and with no need to count calories may eat a full-sized slice as one serving and be getting twice as many calories and other nutrients per serving.

All of the recipes in this book contain a nutritional analysis which specifies how many servings the recipe makes and how many exchanges each serving is. By dividing the loaf of bread, etc. into the number of servings specified, you can easily use these recipes for your diabetic diet.

LOW CALORIE DIETS

Bread, by nature, is a low fat, low calorie food. What makes eating bread "fattening" is putting butter or bologna on it! When you make your own fresh bread, you may find that it has so much flavor that you do not need to put butter on it to make it enjoyable. All of the breads in this book are sugar-free, which may help with weight control more than counting calories. (See "Sugar-Free Diets," page 4.) If you do want to count calories, the nutritional analysis of each recipe will allow you to do so easily.

HOW TO USE THE NUTRITIONAL ANALYSES OF THE RECIPES IN THIS BOOK

Each recipe in this book is followed by a nutritional analysis.* This analysis contains the number of calories, grams of protein, carbohydrate, and fat (total and saturated), milligrams of cholesterol, milligrams of sodium, and grams of fiber per serving and per loaf. Two sets of values per loaf are given if the recipe makes two sizes of loaves. Also included is a "Percent Daily Value" column, which tells what percent, based on a 2000 calorie diet, of your daily requirement of each nutrient is fulfilled by one serving.

If you divide the loaf of bread into the number of servings specified in the recipe, you can use the "per serving" values given to find out, for instance, how many calories a serving of the bread contains. If you cut your bread into a different number of slices, divide the values given for the whole loaf by the number of slices you cut to determine how much of each nutrient one slice contains.

For some of the recipes, such as a sweet roll dough recipe, the nutritional analysis is given for the whole recipe only. If you use this dough to make another recipe, such as cinnamon rolls, add the whole-recipe values for the dough to the values given in the cinnamon roll recipe for the added ingredients, such as raisins, oil, and sweeteners, and divide by the number of rolls you made to get the nutritional values for each roll.

If you are given a choice between optional ingredients in a recipe, the nutritional analysis will be based on the first choice given. If there are significant nutritional differences between the two choices, such as between egg substitutes and eggs, a nutritional analysis will be given for both choices.

For those who are not counting calories and not on diabetic diets, the nutritional analyses may be used in a more general, comparative way. For instance, if you want to increase the amount of fiber in your diet, use the nutritional analyses to compare the grams of fiber per serving for two different kinds of bread when deciding which one to make. You can compare the amount of fat or saturated fat in a doughnut made from one of the recipes in this book to that in a commercial doughnut, and see just how much good you are doing yourself or your family by making your own fresh doughnuts. Use the nutritional analyses as general guidelines to help make wise choices about what you will eat.

---

*The nutritional analyses in this book have been calculated from the nutritional values of foods given in several sources, including *Foods and Nutrition Encyclopedia* by Audrey H. Ensminger, M. E. Ensminger, James E. Kolande, and John R. K. Robinson, M.D., Pegus Press, 1983, *Perspectives In Nutrition* by Gordon M. Wardlaw, Ph.D., R.D., L.D. and Paul M. Insel, Ph.D., Mosby College Publishing, 1990, and information supplied by the producers of several of the food ingredients. Every effort has been made to insure that these analyses are as accurate as possible. However, since they are based on values that were measured from a limited number of samples of the foods involved, they are, by their very nature, approximations.

All About Yeast Breads

What is yeast bread? It is flour and water, and usually a little salt and sweetener. The miracle workers that make these simple ingredients into one of our most delicious foods are yeast, the proper application of heat, and the development of a good structure (usually gluten) of the bread dough.

Yeast is single celled microorganism, and is what makes yeast breads rise and become the light, fluffy, flavorful delights that we expect them to be. The yeast does this by producing carbon dioxide gas, which is trapped in the structure of the bread, and causes it to expand.

Several factors influence this process. The most important is the temperature at which the yeast grows and multiplies. When yeast breads are made by hand, the dough should be kept at about 85-90°F during the rising process, both initially after the dough is made, and after the dough is shaped and put in the pan for the second rise before baking.

The proper temperature of the water used to dissolve the yeast varies depending on the method you are using to make the dough. When making bread by hand or using a mixer, the temperature of the water should be about 115°F because the bread will cool as it kneads. When using a bread machine or food processor, the water should be at or slightly above room temperature, about 80°F, because the bread machine or food processor will heat up the dough slightly as it kneads. The other ingredients that are put into the bread should all be at about room temperature.

There are two almost-foolproof ways to create a cozy place for your yeast bread to rise (or "proof") if you are making it by hand, mixer, or food processor. One is to heat your electric oven to 350°F for 5 minutes, turn it off, and leave the door open until it cools to about 90°F. (A yeast thermometer is an essential tool for checking both the temperature of your rising place and the water used to dissolve the yeast.) Then close the door, and you will have a warm, draft-free rising place for your bread. Or, if you have a gas stove, it is said that the pilot light keeps the inside of the oven at just the right temperature for bread dough to rise.

The second method of keeping your yeast bread at the right temperature during its rising time is to use a microwave oven with multiple power settings. In a microwave, your yeast bread will rise more quickly and save you time, although initially it will take a little experimentation to determine the right setting to use for each microwave oven. To use your microwave to proof your bread, see pages 18 to 19.

In addition to the proper temperature, other factors influence the growth of yeast. One is the availability of food. Most bread recipes contain some type of sugar (usually fruit sugar in this book) to nourish the yeast, although Italian and French breads may not. (In Italian and French breads, the yeast is nourished more slowly as the enzymes in the flour break down some of the starch into sugar.) Acidity influences the growth of the yeast. Yeast prefers slightly acid conditions, but too much acid, such as is encountered when you try to make the dough very sweet using fruit sweeteners, can inhibit the growth of the yeast. Salt also moderates the growth of yeast. Bread made without salt will rise much faster and higher, and may fall during baking if it overproofs (rises too much.)

The gas made by the yeast must be trapped by the bread dough to cause the dough to rise. In breads made with wheat and spelt, and to a lesser degree rye and kamut, the gluten naturally present in the flour is developed into a network of fibers that traps the gas during the kneading process. Kneading causes small molecules of the gluten proteins to form long chains and sheets. This makes the dough feel smooth and elastic, and when you poke your finger into it, it will spring back. The gas made by the yeast is trapped in this gluten structure, and the result is light, fluffy bread.

There are several methods of kneading bread dough to properly develop the gluten structure. The most basic is old fashioned hand kneading. The yeast bread recipes in this book can be made this way if desired; hand kneading is a therapeutic activity if you have the energy for it. If you are interested in making your bread with less effort, you can knead it using a mixer or food processor as described on pages 19 to 20. And of course, a bread machine does all of the kneading automatically, as well as controlling the rising time, maintaining the right temperature, and baking the bread.

If you wish to make gluten-free breads, such as rice, buckwheat, quinoa, or amaranth bread, or breads that contain only a small amount of gluten, such as barley or oat bread, you will have to add something to trap the gas and strengthen the structure of the bread. The most common ingredients to add are guar gum or xanthum gum. Both are soluble fibers that form into chains during kneading. They are not as strong as gluten, so if the dough rises too much, your bread will fall during baking. Other ingredients, such as tapioca flour and eggs, also help to strengthen the structure of gluten-free or low-gluten breads. The structure of these breads is best developed by a mixer or bread machine.

All yeast bread making is based on the handmade bread process, so in order to understand making yeast breads in a bread machine, an understanding of the hand process is valuable. Also, if you wish to make the recipes in this book by hand, you can do so by this process. Or, if you wish to make dough in your bread machine and then bake it into a more conventional shape, you can finish the second rising and baking by this process.

To make yeast bread by hand, begin by combining the water and sweetener called for in the recipe in a bowl. Sprinkle the active dry yeast over the surface of the liquid and allow it to stand for 10 to 15 minutes, or until it bubbles or "proofs." Stir in the salt, oil, and about half of the flour, and beat it until it is elastic. Stir in as much of the remaining flour as you can, and then turn the dough out onto a floured board to knead it. Knead it by pushing on it with the heels of your hands, folding it over, turning it 90°, and the repeating the process over and over for about 10 minutes, gradually adding more flour, until the dough is smooth and elastic. The "feel" of the bread will tell you when enough flour has been added; it will no longer be sticky and will be very resilient. Hand-kneaded bread will absorb a little more flour than called for in most bread machine recipes. Other ingredients, such as nuts and raisins, may be added during this kneading time.

Put the dough in an oiled bowl, and turn it over to oil the other side of the dough. Cover it with plastic wrap or a towel, and allow it to rise in a warm place, such as your oven, as described above, or microwave until it has doubled in volume. In an oven, this will take 45 to 60 minutes for most kinds of breads. In a microwave (this method is described on p. 18-19), it will take about 15 minutes. If quick-rise yeast is used instead of active dry yeast, the rising time will be about ⅓ shorter.

Punch the dough down and form it into a loaf, rolls, or whatever shape you desire. Place it into an oiled pan and allow it to rise until doubled again. If your dough is rising in the oven or a warm spot in your kitchen, the second rise will take less time than the first rise. If you are using the microwave method of proofing your dough (described on p.18-19), the second rise will take about 15 minutes. To tell when gluten-containing dough is ready to bake, poke it gently with your finger. If it does not spring back, it is ready. Gluten-free or non-gluten doughs should be judged visually by looking at their size. It is better to bake them when they are only 1¾ times their original volume than to let them overproof, or they may collapse during baking.

If you are proofing the bread in your oven, take it out when it has risen enough. Preheat the oven to 350°F for most loaf breads or 375°F for most rolls. Bake from 15 to 20 minutes for rolls. Light, fluffy, gluten-containing breads will take 45 minutes to an hour to bake. Dense whole grain, low-gluten, or non-gluten breads can take over an hour to bake. The bread is done when it is brown and pulls away from the sides of the pan. To keep the crust from getting soggy, remove the bread from the pan immediately after baking. For light, fluffy, gluten-containing breads, if you tap the bottom of the loaf and it sounds hollow, it is done. The more dense breads may not sound hollow, but should be well browned. If sweet breads brown too rapidly during baking, cover them with a piece of foil partway through the baking time.

Most experts recommend letting your bread cool off before you cut it and eat it. However, around our house, it smells so good that some of the little people can't wait that long. I have found that if I use a good bread knife and a gentle sawing motion to cut it, I can cut it immediately without smashing the loaf, although the cut edge may not be as nice as if it had completely cooled off before I cut it. You may be able to purchase a good bread knife, such as a Henckels, in a discount store, as I did, for a fraction of the price that they sell for in cooking catalogues or stores. My knife is probably not "top of the line," but it works very well.

Homemade bread keeps best when stored at room temperature or in the freezer. It gets stale more quickly in the refrigerator. Always let your bread cool completely before storing it. A good, economical way to store bread is in a plastic bag on the kitchen counter. The crust will soften in a plastic bag. Some people use paper or waxed paper bags to store bread if they want the crust to stay crisp. Bread boxes are highly recommended for storing bread. My experience with them has been very positive. You do not need to use plastic bags when you store bread in a bread box. If you want to see how bread keeps in a bread box before buying one, store some rolls in a metal pan with a snug-fitting lid. The King Arthur Flour Baker's Catalogue (see "Sources," p. 235) carries an excellent bread box.

Homemade bread can be a budget stretcher. Some family members, who might balk at having soup for dinner every few days, think soup and freshly made bread is a great treat, and look forward to soup-and-bread nights. Such meals are much more in line with the USDA's new food guidelines than traditional meals as well. And if you are cooking for a special diet and can find commercial bread you can eat, it may cost over $3 for a small loaf, so for special breads, the money you save by making your own can really add up over a period of time.

Homemade yeast breads are one of life's most basic simple pleasures. May this book introduce you to the enjoyment of easily making your own.

All About Quick Breads

What is quick bread? Like yeast bread, it is flour and water, and usually a little salt and sweetener, but it is leavened by the chemical reaction between baking soda and an acid ingredient rather than by the action of yeast. Because there is no need for yeast to grow and multiply, it is baked immediately after mixing, and therefore can be made more quickly than yeast bread.

When baking soda is mixed with an acid ingredient in a liquid environment, carbon dioxide gas is immediately formed. It is trapped in the batter or dough and will be baked as little bubbles into the final product. There are many different acid ingredients that you can use. Cream of tartar and vitamin C crystals are two dry acid ingredients. Baking powder consists of an acid ingredient plus baking soda and some starch (usually cornstarch) to keep the baking soda and acid apart and dry until you are ready to bake. Quick breads can be made with a wide variety of liquid acid ingredients, such as fruit juices, vinegar, or buttermilk.

There are many kinds of non-yeast bread products besides just breads: muffins, pancakes, and crackers are just a few of them. If you need to make these items for use on an allergy diet, refer to *Allergy Cooking With Ease,* described on the last page of this book.

There are several bread machines now on the market that have a quick bread or cake cycle that can make yeast-free bread for you from start to finish. As with yeast breads, understanding the process of making quick breads by hand will help you use these machines.

To make non-yeast breads conventionally, combine the dry ingredients in a bowl. These consist of flour, salt, spices, and dry leavening ingredients, such as baking powder, baking soda, cream of tartar, or vitamin C crystals. If you must avoid baking powder because of allergy to the starch component, which is usually corn, you can use baking soda in conjunction with an acid ingredient, such as vitamin C crystals, cream of tartar, citrus juice, vinegar, buttermilk, or acid fruit juices. Combine the liquid ingredients in a separate bowl or cup. These include water, oil, fruit juice, fruit purees, eggs, liquid acid leavening ingredients, etc.

It is very important to preheat your oven and to oil and flour your baking pans before you mix the liquid and dry ingredients together, because the chemical reaction that produces leavening begins immediately upon mixing and may be finished before you get the bread into the oven if there is any delay. When everything is ready, and you do not think the phone is going to ring, quickly stir the liquid ingredients into the dry ingredients. It is more important to be quick than thorough about this; if some lumps or dry spots remain, do not worry. Overmixing is much more likely to cause problems with quick breads than undermixing. Put the batter into the prepared pan and bake, usually at 350°F, for 35 minutes to an hour, depending on the type of bread. To test non-yeast breads for doneness, insert a wooden toothpick into the center of the loaf. If it comes out dry, the bread is done. The loaf should also be nicely browned.

Quick breads made without eggs or fruit purees can be quite fragile. It is important to cool these breads completely on a rack before slicing them. But if you make a very sturdy bread, such as banana bread, go ahead and enjoy it as soon as it comes out of the oven or bread machine.

I usually store quick breads in a plastic bag at room temperature or in the freezer. Some of the fruit-containing breads can be quite moist, and I may put them in the refrigerator to prevent mold growth if they are not getting eaten quickly. Quick breads do not seem to get stale in the refrigerator as readily as yeast breads do.

For those on yeast-free diets, quick breads are a very important part of the diet. For others, they provide variety, and the fruit-containing quick breads and cakes make great desserts.

Let's Make It Easy: Equipment to Help You

We have many advantages our grandmothers did not have when it comes to making bread. Instead of having to use short-lived compressed yeast, we have very reliable active dry yeast. We can make our bread with appliances we already have, such as our mixers and food processors, and use our microwave ovens to cause it to rise quickly. Or, we can use a bread machine to do everything but measure the ingredients for us. Today breadmaking is a joy rather than a chore.

This chapter will explore some of the appliances that can help you make bread quickly and effortlessly.

MICROWAVE OVENS

As mentioned on page 12, you can use your microwave oven to warm your bread and cause it to rise much more quickly than it normally would. Using a food processor and microwave, you can make homemade bread in just two hours. Your microwave must have an adjustable power setting. Most microwave ovens made now can be set at a low enough power to warm your bread dough without killing the yeast. However, you will have to experiment a little to find the power level and time that works best for your microwave.

To use the microwave method of proofing your bread dough, put the kneaded dough in a glass bowl and place it in the microwave. Put an 8-oz. glass of water in one corner of the microwave oven. As a beginning point, set the power level to 10%. Microwave for 2 minutes. If the dough feels hot (or stick your yeast thermometer into the dough - it should never be over 112°F), allow the dough to rest in the oven for four minutes. If it does not feel hot, but rather just cool to lukewarm, microwave it for an additional minute and allow it to rest for three minutes. Then microwave it again for 2 or 3 minutes (the same amount of time that you used before) and allow it to rest for 6 or 7 minutes in the microwave. At the end of this time, the dough should feel comfortably warm, have doubled in volume, and an indentation should remain when poked with your finger. If it is not warm or has not doubled, try gradually increasing the power setting you use, but never go above 30%. If you use glass baking pans, the dough can be proofed in the microwave after shaping the loaf also.

If your dough felt hot after the first two minutes of microwaving on 10% power and does not rise properly, you should use the oven method, pages 11 to 12, for proofing your dough.

Some microwave oven instruction manuals and cookbooks contain recipes for baking yeast breads in the microwave. I have not found this method to be satisfactory, mainly because microwave oven baked breads do not brown.

MIXERS

Any electric mixer can do at least part of the kneading required to make yeast bread, and heavy-duty mixers can do all of the kneading for you. There are a number of mixers on the market that do a great job of doing all of the kneading by themselves. Kitchen Aid mixers are strong enough to develop gluten properly without any help from you, and can make dough for two loaves of bread per batch. They can be used for two batches in a row before you must allow your machine a 45 minute cool down period.

Kenwood mixers have a very powerful motor and a thermal overload protector, so can be used for as many batches of bread dough in a row as desired. The models with 7-quart bowls can be used to make dough for up to four loaves of bread at a time. You may have to stop and scrape the bowl during the initial mixing to get all of the flour to mix in efficiently.

Bosch mixers also have a powerful motor and a thermal overload protector, so they can be used to make an unlimited number of batches of dough consecutively. The large Bosch Universal mixer can make dough for five loaves of bread at a time. These mixers mix the flour in very efficiently and "clean the bowl" without any assistance.

There are several advantages of using a mixer to make bread. One is that by using a large, heavy-duty mixer you can make several loaves at once and store them in your freezer to use as needed. Another advantage is that mixer-made breads have an excellent texture. Because you have an opportunity to check the consistency of the dough by hand, any variations in the amount of flour required because of humidity, flour quality, etc., can be corrected for.

See pages 44 to 45 and 50 for instructions on making yeast breads with a mixer.

FOOD PROCESSORS

A food processor is equipment that many of us already own that can be used to make yeast bread dough with gluten-containing flours. Food processors knead bread dough very quickly. In one minute they achieve excellent gluten development. You can use most processors to knead dough for only one loaf of bread at a time. The opportunity to check the dough by hand allows for the correction of any problems due to variations in the ingredients or weather. The texture of the bread is excellent.

For instructions on using your food processor to make yeast breads, see page 41.

BREAD MACHINES

Bread machines have revolutionized the lives of those of us who must make all of our bread ourselves because of our special diets. All we have to do is measure the ingredients and push a few buttons, and in a few hours we have bread! Several years ago, I had a bread baking day about every two weeks, baked six to ten loaves of various kinds of bread, and stocked up the freezer for the next two weeks. I enjoyed the feel of the dough and the aesthetic experience of making bread myself and was not an easy convert to bread machine baking, but now I could not live without my bread machines. They get as much use as my washer and dryer. For those of us on special diets, a bread machine is not a luxury item, but rather, an essential time and energy saving appliance like a dishwasher or a clothes washer. To go back to making bread by hand now would be almost like digging out my grandmother's old washing board and tub!

BREAD MACHINE FEATURES

There are many factors to consider when choosing a bread machine. Each bread machine has its own assets and drawbacks. Our needs and budgets are different, so there is no one machine that is best for every home baker. Some of the features that you should consider when making this important purchase are price, pan shape and size, viewing window, ease of keeping the machine clean, delayed cycle timer, programmability, the cycles the machine offers, the cool down feature, and the power saver feature.

PRICE: This is probably the first factor that comes to mind when you are thinking about buying a bread machine. There are several economical models on the market now that do a great job of making ordinary breads without all the "bells and whistles" of the luxury machines. Also, most bread machines go on sale occasionally, so it is worth your while to shop around for a good price. By shopping the sales, I purchased a 1-lb. Mr. Loaf machine by Seiko at Walmart for $86. Consider all of the features below and decide which of them you really need before you spend a lot of money on a machine that has features you may rarely use.

PAN SHAPE AND SIZE: Most bread machines make either 1 lb. or 1½ lb. loaves, although there are a few that can make 2 lb. loaves on the market now. Since it is so easy to make bread with a bread machine and bread is best when freshly made, an individual or small family may be kept in bread adequately by a 1-lb. machine. I often run my machines more than once in a day, which is always a possibility with a smaller machine. For a large family, a large machine may be more practical.

Bread machine pans are most often vertically rectangular, but can also be round or horizontally rectangular. Some people prefer round pans because you can have more variety in what your bread slices look like. If you slice the loaf horizontal-

ly, you can have round or half-circle slices. If you slice it vertically, you get normal looking slices. I feel that for making some
of the more unusual types of breads that require assistance in
the mixing and kneading parts of the cycle, machines with
round pans need less help from me, and I like the machine to
do as much of the work as possible.

Machines with horizontally rectangular pans produce
loaves that look almost like store-bought, both as whole loaves
and as slices. Machines with vertically rectangular pans produce
square or rectangular slices. Diabetics may find bread from
machines with rectangular pans easier to divide into a certain
number of equal-sized servings for portion control than bread
from round pans.

VIEWING WINDOW OR DOME: This is a good
feature to have because it is helpful to keep an eye on how your
bread is doing, especially the first time you use a new recipe.
Seeing what was going on has kept the dough from over-rising
and running down over the edge of the pan and onto the heat-
ing coil of the machine more than once for me! But a viewing
window is not an absolutely essential feature. If your machine
does not have a window, you can lift the lid and take a few brief
peeks to see what is happening. I have never had bread come
out underdone or any of the other disasters that the manufacturers predict happen as a result of peeking into the machine.

EASE OF KEEPING THE MACHINE CLEAN:
There is a wide range of variability in how easy bread machines
are to keep clean. Some bread machine pans have holes in the
bottom. The pan must be seated in the machine with the rubber gasket in place before you add ingredients to it. With this
type of machine, it is easy to dribble a little oil onto the outside
of the pan or the inside of the machine, or get other ingredients
in the bottom of the machine. Other machines, which are easier to keep clean, have pans that you remove to add the ingredients. And still other machines have crumb trays at the bottom
and removable lids. I personally would choose a machine that
worked well, even if it were not easy to keep clean, over one that
was easier to keep clean but did not do what I wanted it to do,
but this is an area where your personal neatness preference must

help you decide which machine you prefer.

DELAYED CYCLE TIMER: A timer is a useful feature to have if you want to have bread freshly baked for breakfast or when you will be away from home. If your lifestyle involves a lot of time away from home, this can be an important feature for you. Many machines with timers are called programmable, but this may just mean that you can program what time you want your bread to be done, not that you have the control over the cycles that truly programmable machines, described below, give you. When deciding whether to get a machine with this feature, let your lifestyle and your budget be your guide.

YEAST DISPENSER: Some machines have a separate compartment to add the yeast to, and the machine adds it to the dough after the cycle has begun. This can be an advantage when using your machine on the timer because there is no way that the yeast can get wet before it should. However, if you add the liquid ingredients to the machine first and put the yeast in a small well on top of the flour (even if you normally add ingredients to your machine in the opposite order), the yeast will stay dry without this feature.

PROGRAMMABILITY: If you want to make a variety of non-wheat breads, this is a very important feature for you to consider. In a non-programmable machine, you have one or a few set cycles to choose from. Wheat breads fit these cycles quite well; most of the spelt breads, kamut bread, and some rye breads can also be made using them. But if you wish to make some of the "variety" spelt-based breads, oat, barley, quinoa, amaranth, buckwheat, egg-free rice, or a number of other types of bread, you must have control over the final rising and baking times of the cycle to produce an acceptable loaf of bread.

There are two programmable machines on the market at the time of this writing. Since most of the questions I hear about bread machines are asked by allergy patients wondering how well a bread machine will meet their needs, these two machines will be discussed in detail here. For detailed descriptions of other bread machines, refer to *The Bread Machine Magic Book of Helpful Hints* by Linda Rehberg and Lois Conway.

The first programmable machine to come out was the Zojirushi Home Bakery, model number BBCC-S15. Its list price is $350, although it often sells for about $300. It is available mostly in specialty cooking stores and catalogues. This machine is great for experimenting because on the "homemade menu" cycle you can watch the dough and press a button to advance it to the next part of the cycle when it appears ready. (This makes the use of quick-rise yeast possible with non-wheat flours.) You can set any part of the cycle to the time desired as you run the machine, and can then store your special cycle in the machine's memory immediately after it is completed. However, only one special cycle program can be stored in the machine's memory, so if you plan to make several types of bread which use different cycles, you will have to be at home and set your kitchen timer to push the button that advances the machine to the next part of the cycle several times while the machine is running. Also, because the machine does not knead very vigorously, the flour must be added gradually during the initial mixing, and this machine requires more assistance from you during mixing than other machines do. I suspect because of this machine's less vigorous kneading, neither I nor others I have asked in other parts of the country have been able to make whole grain spelt bread with excellent texture in this machine, although the spelt bread it makes is adequate. (It does make very good wheat breads, though.) Zojirushi machines have an excellent reputation for not needing service. This machine makes 1½ lb. vertically rectangular loaves. It has a jam cycle and a cake cycle that can be used for quick breads.

The other programmable machine currently on the market is the Welbilt Multi-logic Bread Bakery, model number ABM-150R. Its list price is $289, although Sears regularly sells it for $229 and occasionally has it on sale even cheaper. It is available in department and discount stores as well as in cooking stores. The initial kneading and rising times cannot be changed; however, the second knead, second rise, and baking times, which are the critical times, can be set by simply pushing buttons before the cycle begins. Therefore, there is no need to be home and push buttons while the machine is running even if you make a different type of bread using a different cycle each time you bake. The motor is powerful and vigorous enough to mix in all of the flour if it is added to the machine at one time, usually without any assistance from you. Also, the more strenuous kneading this machine does yields a texture in the bread that is as good as handmade bread, even for whole grain spelt bread. Welbilt machines are very reliable; I have used mine anywhere from several times to dozens of times per week for over 1½ years and have never had any problems with it. This machine makes 1½ lb. round loaves and has a quick bread or cake cycle.

DOUGH CYCLE: A bread machine with a dough cycle feature makes the dough and allows it to rise, and then stops the machine before baking so you can shape and bake the dough as you desire. Some of the cheaper machines claim to have a dough cycle, but what they really have is a buzzer that tells you when to remove the dough from the machine if you do not want it to be baked. If you are not at home or are not paying attention to your machine, it may bake your dough before you notice it. With any machine, you can set a timer to remind you to stop the machine before it bakes, but a dough cycle that turns the machine off for you is a very useful feature to have if you want to have dough ready to make into rolls or pizza for dinner when you are not going to be home in the afternoon.

QUICK YEAST CYCLE: A quick yeast cycle allows you to use quick-rise yeast to make wheat breads more quickly than the regular cycles on the bread machine, or to make bread with regular active dry yeast in a shorter amount of time. This cycle is useful for making a limited number of non-wheat yeast breads with regular active dry yeast because the second rising time is shorter than in the regular cycles. However, the second rise is still too long for most of the non-wheat flours that require a programmable cycle. This cycle is good for people in a hurry, but again, your budget may be a deciding factor on this feature.

QUICK BREAD (NON-YEAST) OR CAKE CYCLE:

This cycle is essential if you are allergic to yeast or want to make non-yeast quick breads or cakes in your bread machine. If you rarely make cake or non-yeast breads, this may not be an essential cycle for you because quick breads are easy to make by hand. When deciding on this feature, let your dietary needs, your budget, and how much you like cakes be your guide.

WHOLE GRAIN CYCLE: If you plan to make a lot of 100% whole wheat bread, this can be a useful cycle on some machines. But most machines have a fairly long standard yeast bread cycle, with quite a bit of time devoted to kneading and a long second rise, so the whole grain cycle does not produce results that are substantially different from the standard cycle. If you are considering buying a bread machine for its whole grain cycle, consult the instruction booklet or the manufacturer for the times the machine spends on kneading and the second rise for both the standard and whole grain cycles and compare them to see if they are much different.

FRENCH BREAD CYCLE: This cycle is for dough that is low in fat and sugar and takes longer to rise. If you think that French and Italian breads should be long, thin, crispy-crusted loaves rather than bread machine pan shaped loaves, you may prefer to make French bread by using the dough cycle, shaping the loaves on baking sheets, brushing the crust with a wash (see the recipe on p. 129) to make it crispy, and baking it in the oven. You can produce much better French and Italian bread by this method than by purchasing a machine for its french bread cycle.

RAISIN BREAD CYCLE: A raisin bread cycle is usually a fairly standard cycle with a "beep" to tell you when to add raisins or nuts to your bread machine so they do not get mashed by the full kneading cycle. Once you know how long your machine kneads on the standard cycle, you can set your kitchen timer for 5 to 10 minutes before the last kneading time should be finished when you start the machine, and add the raisins or nuts when the timer rings. Therefore, while helpful, this is not an essential bread machine feature.

SWEET BREAD CYCLE: A sweet bread cycle allows the dough more rising time and bakes it at a lower temperature than the standard cycle does. Even when the sweet bread cycle is used, I still find that the crust of sweet breads baked in the machine is darker than I prefer. Instead of using the sweet bread cycle to make sweet breads, I use the dough cycle, shape the dough imaginatively, and bake the bread in the oven, where it is easier to control how dark the crust will get.

CRUST DARKNESS CONTROL: Some experienced bread machine bakers consider this feature essential. I personally almost always leave the darkness control on "medium" and really do not use it. When I have tried using "light" for sweet breads, the crust has still come out too dark. So this is not a feature that I would pay extra money for, although if the machine that you plan to get for other reasons has it, it is certainly not a drawback.

COOL DOWN OR KEEP WARM FEATURE AT THE END OF THE CYCLE: If you tend to get busy with other things and forget about your bread machine, or if you want to leave home while it is running, a cool down feature is a very helpful feature to have. It will keep your bread from getting soggy if you do not remove it from the machine immediately. A keep warm feature keeps your bread warm and, on most machines, also keeps it from getting soggy if you do not remove it from the machine as soon as it finishes baking.

MOTOR NOISE AND KNEADING VIGOR: The amount of noise your bread machine makes and the vigor with which it kneads the bread are usually two sides of the same coin. The machines that knead more vigorously produce good gluten development and excellent texture and tend to be more noisy. The machines that are the quietest may make inferior bread. So unless you plan to routinely make bread for breakfast using the delayed cycle timer and your bed is on the other side of your kitchen wall, I would not consider quietness an important feature. Even the noisiest bread machines make less noise than most microwave ovens or dishwashers, and they only make it when they are kneading.

POWER SAVER FEATURE: Some bread machines have a backup system that keeps them functioning during short (10 or 15 minute) power outages. If your machine does not have this feature, and the power outage occurs early in the cycle, you may be able to re-start the machine. Or, you can pull the dough out of the machine, let it rise in a bread pan, and bake it in the oven. If you live in an area that has frequent short power outages, this feature may be important to you.

THE CHOICE is yours. At an allergy cooking class I was recently asked, "Do you have any recommendations for people who are on a special diet and don't want to spend a lot of time cooking?" My immediate reply was, "Get a bread machine." If you are on a special diet, a bread machine can save you a lot of time and energy. When you begin planning to buy a bread machine, get information about the machines you are considering from the manufacturers. Or go to stores and look at bread machines and the instruction booklets that come with them. Shop around for sales, and get the machine that best serves your needs for the lowest price. Then enjoy your home-made bread and the time you do not have to spend making it.

The Building Blocks of Bread

Just as we are what we eat, our bread is as good as what we put into it. One of the greatest advantages of making your own bread is that you control what goes into it. You can put in the freshest, most wholesome ingredients and leave out the preservatives and chemicals that are found in many commercial breads. Knowledge of the ingredients you can use to build your bread and using the best ingredients available will help you turn out delicious, nutritious loaves every time.

FLOURS

Flour is the most basic building block of bread. For all yeast breads, but especially if you are using a bread machine, it is essential that you use good quality flour. For bread machine bread, it is also essential that you measure accurately if you want your bread to turn out well every time.

Flour does not need to be sifted before measuring. Simply stir it to loosen it, lightly spoon it into your measuring cup, and level it off with a straight-edged knife or spatula. Resist the temptation to pack flour into the cup, or a heavy, dry loaf of bread may result.

Even with the best flour, there can be many variables, such as the moisture and gluten content. When making bread by hand these variables are corrected for by adding flour until the bread "feels right." With a bread machine, you will learn to judge the bread by how it looks and by reaching into the machine and seeing how it feels. "Right" for bread machine bread is usually softer than "right" for bread made by hand. Also, for some types of flour, such as rye, the right texture of the dough is quite sticky.

Many people wish to grind their own flour from whole grains in order to make fresher, better tasting, more economical, and more nutritious bread. Home ground flours are delicious, but can be more variable than commercial flour because we cannot test the flour for gluten content, etc., before we use it. If you are a beginning bread maker, or are just getting used

to using a bread machine, it may be best to start with high quality, reliable commercial flour until you learn the right feel of the
dough. Then, after you have gained some experience, you will
be able to judge the dough and compensate for variations in
your home ground flour by using slightly more or less flour or
water.

THE KINDS OF FLOUR USED IN THE RECIPES IN THIS BOOK INCLUDE:

BREAD FLOUR is wheat flour made from high-gluten
wheat. The higher gluten content of this flour makes it perfect
for bread machine breads. The bran and germ have been
removed from bread flour, and some brands are bleached and
bromated. King Arthur Special flour (see "Sources," page 236)
is an excellent bread flour that has not been chemically treated.
If you live in an area of the country where you cannot get King
Arthur flour easily, beware that not all bread flour works equal-
ly well. One national brand I used usually worked well, but
then I got a couple of bags that made flat-topped, fallen loaves
of bread until I began adding vital gluten to the loaves I made
with it. If you wish to use a national brand of bread flour, I have
found Pillsbury's bread flour yields consistently good results.

ALL PURPOSE FLOUR is a refined wheat flour that
is lower in gluten content than bread flour. It is used in the
quick bread recipes in this book. It may be used for making
yeast breads by hand, but will require that more flour be added
to the recipe than if bread flour is used.

WHOLE WHEAT BREAD FLOUR is whole wheat
flour that has been ground from hard red spring or winter
wheat and is higher in gluten than most whole wheat flours.
(Graham flour is whole wheat flour ground from low-gluten
wheat.) If you use whole wheat bread flour in your bread
machine rather than regular whole wheat flour, it will make
breads that rise well even though they are 100% whole grain.
Arrowhead Mills produces an excellent whole wheat bread
flour.

WHOLE WHEAT ALL PURPOSE FLOUR is whole wheat flour that is lower in gluten than whole wheat bread flour. It is used in quick breads in this book.

WHITE WHOLE WHEAT FLOUR is milled from hard white wheat. It is lighter in flavor and color than whole wheat bread flour, and so may be more acceptable to people who are not whole grain enthusiasts. It makes excellent bread. King Arthur Flour offers a great white whole wheat flour. (See "Sources, p. 236.)

GLUTEN FLOUR is a refined wheat flour that is about 40 to 50% gluten. It is very high in protein, and is often used by hypoglycemics. It can be used to "fix" low quality flours by adding more gluten to the recipe. Use about ¼ c. gluten flour and ¾ c. of the other flour for each cup of flour called for in the recipe.

VITAL GLUTEN is refined wheat flour that has had the starch removed and is almost all gluten. It is commonly used to "fix" low quality flours and to make dense breads rise better. However, if you use it to make non-wheat breads rise better, the bread will no longer be wheat-free, because vital gluten comes from wheat. If you are using it to improve other flours, use 2 to 4 tsp. for a small loaf of bread and up to 2 tbsp. for a large loaf. Vital gluten is not used in the recipes in this book because I have found that if you use good quality flour, the bread turns out well without it, and I prefer starting with good flour to trying to "fix" bad flour.

WHOLE SPELT FLOUR: Spelt is a grain that is closely related to wheat and is higher in gluten than wheat. Spelt makes excellent breads, but I have found more variability in spelt flour than for any other kind of flour. Even the best spelt flour can vary from bag to bag, so always test the consistency of the dough as described on p.55 when you start your bread. The only brand of spelt flour I have used that consistently produces excellent bread is Purity Foods spelt flour. (See "Sources," p. 237.) Purity Foods flour is milled from a European strain of spelt that is higher in protein and gluten than most spelt. All of their flour is organic. All of the spelt recipes in this book were developed using Purity Foods flour.

WHITE SPELT FLOUR is whole spelt flour that has been sifted, removing the fibrous elements of the grain, but not bleached, bromated, or enriched like refined wheat flour usually is. It is available only from Purity Foods. (See "Sources," p. 237.) It is the best flour for making non-wheat breads in a bread machine, and produces light, fluffy breads that are almost impossible to distinguish from wheat breads. As with whole spelt flour, always test the consistency of the dough as described on p.55 when you start your bread to compensate for variations in the flour.

KAMUT FLOUR: Kamut is another grain that is closely related to wheat. Although the gluten structure it forms in yeast bread is not as strong as wheat's structure, it still produces very good bread. It is golden yellow in color and has a flavor very similar to wheat. Kamut breads made without a bread machine need only one rising time. After you make the dough, shape it and put it in loaf pans immediately, and bake it after it rises once.

RYE FLOUR is a gluten-containing flour, although it is lower in gluten than wheat. Whole grain rye flour produces dense but very flavorful breads. I have occasionally had difficulty with rye flour from health food store bulk bins making bread that did not rise properly. Arrowhead Mills rye flour produces consistently good bread.

WHITE RYE FLOUR is rye flour with the bran and germ removed. Lighter bread can be made from white rye flour than from whole rye flour. It is also a good choice for those on low fiber diets. An excellent white rye flour is available from King Arthur Flour. (See "Sources, p. 236.)

BROWN RICE FLOUR is milled from the whole rice grain, and contains the rice polish, bran, and germ. It is a gluten-free flour, and is acceptable on celiac diets. Bread made from rice flour usually contains ingredients to strengthen the structure, such as eggs. Egg-free rice bread can be made by hand or in a programmable bread machine by using guar gum to strengthen the structure of the bread.

WHITE RICE FLOUR is milled from rice that has been polished, so the fibrous portions of the grain have been removed. White rice flour is a good bread ingredient for those on low fiber diets.

BARLEY FLOUR is a low-gluten flour. If you wish to make bread from only barley flour in a bread machine, you will need a programmable machine, because the structure of barley bread is fragile. If it rises for a standard amount of time, it will collapse during baking.

OAT FLOUR is also a low-gluten flour. As with barley, a programmable machine is necessary to make good oat-only bread. Oats are an excellent source of soluble fiber.

CORN MEAL gives bread an interesting texture and a sweet flavor. It is gluten-free, and is acceptable on celiac diets.

SOY FLOUR is ground from soybeans. It is very high in protein, and may be used to increase the protein content of breads. It is acceptable on celiac diets.

CAROB POWDER is a substitute for cocoa on allergy diets. Added to Pumpernickel Bread, it gives a rich brown color.

AMARANTH FLOUR is a non-grain flour that is quite useful to people who are allergic to all grains. It is very nutritious and high in protein, but has more problems with stickiness than any other kind of flour I have worked with. However, since there have been times in my life when it was the only flour I could eat, I persisted in using it, and if my bread came out sticky, I sliced and toasted it. Amaranth flour makes very dense bread. Purchase it from a store that either has a high turnover or refrigerates its flour and store it in the refrigerator or freezer at home, or it will develop a strong flavor.

QUINOA FLOUR is another non-grain flour. Quinoa is related to beets and spinach. It is high in protein and calcium and is very nutritious. It has a distinctive flavor, and is best in breads that contain fruit, which moderates the flavor. Quinoa breads are very dense.

BUCKWHEAT FLOUR is a non-grain flour. Dark buckwheat flour is ground from roasted buckwheat groats. Arrowhead Mills produces an excellent dark buckwheat flour that consistently makes good bread. White buckwheat flour is ground from unroasted groats. Commercial white buckwheat flour can vary tremendously from bag to bag, even from the same source. White buckwheat flour is often home ground. If you wish to make bread from white buckwheat flour, make a loaf or two of regular buckwheat bread with Arrowhead Mills flour first to gain experience with what the consistency of buckwheat bread dough should be like. Then, make bread with white buckwheat flour using the same recipe and, if necessary, adding more flour to reach the same consistency. You can often substitute white buckwheat flour for dark buckwheat flour in equal amounts.

TAPIOCA FLOUR, also called tapioca starch or tapioca starch flour, is a white starch that is an excellent addition to gluten-free or low-gluten breads. It strengthens the structure of these breads and allows them to rise better.

ARROWROOT is a white starch that looks much like cornstarch and may be used in place of tapioca flour to strengthen the structure of gluten-free breads.

POTATO FLOUR: Unlike tapioca, potato flour and potato starch are not the same thing. The recipes in this book use potato flour, which is a less refined flour, rather than potato starch. Potato flour is a useful addition to gluten-free rice breads. Bob's Red Mill offers a good potato flour. (See "Sources," p. 236.)

LEAVENING INGREDIENTS

There are several varieties of yeast that you can use to make bread, either by hand or in your bread machine. Non-yeast breads are leavened by a variety of ingredients. The leavening ingredients used in this book include:

ACTIVE DRY YEAST: Active dry yeast is yeast that has been freeze-dried to retain its activity. An expiration date is usually stamped on the package, and the yeast should be good until that date if you store it in the refrigerator after opening it. Active dry yeast is available in ¼ oz. (2¼ tsp.) packets or 4 oz. jars in most grocery stores. Also, you can purchase it in 1 lb. bags and store the yeast in your freezer. Do not thaw and refreeze this yeast, but rather occasionally take out a small amount to use within a few weeks and keep it in a jar in the refrigerator. I have had consistently good results using Red Star Yeast in my bread machines.

INSTANT, BREAD MACHINE, OR QUICK-RISE YEAST: Although the recipes in this book do not call for these types of yeast, you may wish to use them in your bread machine. If you are making bread with a good gluten structure, you can add the same amount of these types of yeast as of active dry yeast to produce a higher, lighter loaf. (But the first time you do this with each recipe, watch your bread machine to make sure the dough is not going to run over the edge of the pan.) Or you may wish to decrease the amount of yeast used by about ¼ to ½ to produce a more normal sized loaf. Quick-rise yeast can be used to make wheat-containing breads more quickly using the quick yeast cycle on some bread machines, or to make breads that rise more quickly by hand. These types of yeast are not recommended for most of the non-wheat bread machine breads because their gluten structure is more fragile; if these yeasts are used, the bread may over-rise and then collapse during baking.

BAKING POWDER: The quick breads in this book are leavened by baking powder, either alone or with baking soda. Baking powder is used in all of the bread machine quick bread recipes in this book because it can withstand the longer mixing times that the machines use without exhausting all of its leavening power. Baking powder is a combination of baking soda, an acid ingredient, and a starch. Some baking powders contain aluminum, which probably should be avoided for good health. Rumford baking powder is aluminum-free and contains cornstarch. If you must avoid cornstarch because of a corn allergy, Featherweight baking powder contains potato starch.

BAKING SODA: In handmade quick breads, baking soda may be used with a variety of acid ingredients to produce leavening. If you are making bread with baking soda and an acid ingredient rather than baking powder, be sure to work quickly so the leavening activity is not over before the bread goes into the oven. (See pages 16 to 17.) Baking soda is used along with baking powder in some of this book's bread machine quick bread recipes that contain acidic fruits.

SWEETNERS

FRUIT JUICE CONCENTRATES, which are purchased frozen, are used extensively in the recipes in this book. Yeast grows best when it has some sugar to nourish it, and the fruit sugar in fruit juice concentrates is a healthy food for both yeast and people. If you bake bread often, you may wish to keep a can of apple juice concentrate in your refrigerator so it is always thawed and ready to use in breads.

Many of the recipes in this book use apple juice concentrate as a sweetener. If you are allergic to apples, you can use another fruit juice concentrate, such as pineapple juice concentrate. Or, you can use a juice, such as white grape juice. To use a juice (not a concentrate), use four times the amount of juice as the amount of apple juice concentrate the recipe calls for, and decrease the water by three times the volume of apple juice concentrate the recipe calls for. For example, if you want to use white grape juice to make a 1½ lb. loaf of White Bread, p. 61, you would use 1 c. of grape juice (this amount is four times the ¼ c. of apple juice concentrate called for) and ⅛ c. water (this is the ⅞ c. water called for minus ¾ c., which is three times the amount of apple juice concentrate called for.) The total amount of liquid must stay the same. In this example, for the original recipe:

> ¼ c. apple juice concentrate
> + ⅞ c. water
> _____
> 1⅛ c. liquid.

After making the substitution:

> 1 c. white grape juice
> + ⅛ c. water
> _____
> 1⅛ c. liquid.

The total amount of water plus fruit juice used in the recipe is the same before and after the substitution.

FRUIT SWEET™, GRAPE SWEET™, AND LIQUID FRUIT SOURCE™ are more concentrated fruit juice sweeteners than frozen fruit juice concentrates. Fruit Sweet™ is a combination of peach, pear, and pineapple juice concentrates. Grape Sweet™ is made from grape juice concentrate. Fruit Source™ is made from grape juice concentrate and rice syrup. All three are useful in sweet breads where more sweetness is desired than can be added with regular fruit juice concentrates. If too much of these sweeteners is used in yeast breads, the acid can inhibit the growth of the yeast.

GRANULAR FRUIT SOURCE™ is a crystallized form of Fruit Source™ and is useful in making Cinnamon Rolls, Monkey Bread, and other treats where it is nice to have a sugar substitute that you can sprinkle.

DATE SUGAR is ground dried dates. It is useful both in sweet bread doughs and as a sweetener you can sprinkle, such as in Cinnamon Rolls.

HONEY is a sweeter-tasting and more concentrated sweetener than the fruit sweeteners above. It also has a more profound effect on blood sugar levels, and may not be tolerated by hypoglycemics and allergy patients with candidiasis. It can be used as an alternative ingredient to fruit sweeteners in some of the recipes in this book where more sweetness may be desired.

FATS

OIL is used in minimal amounts in most of the bread recipes in this book. Fats make bread tender and keep it from becoming stale rapidly.

LECITHIN: Liquid lecithin is included as an optional ingredient in most of the recipes in this book because it is very effective at keeping bread from getting dry and adds moistness to the bread more effectively than oil. It is also said to be a dough conditioner and promote higher rising, although I have not noticed that it makes much difference in this regard. Liquid lecithin is very sticky, but can be easily measured by measuring the oil first and then using the same spoon to measure the lecithin.

MISCELLANEOUS INGREDIENTS

SALT is a very important ingredient in yeast breads. It moderates the growth of the yeast, and prevents overproofing which can lead to the bread collapsing when it is baked. It strengthens the gluten structure of the bread by inhibiting enzymes in the flour that break gluten down. Salt also adds flavor to bread. A few salt-free recipes made with wheat and spelt are included in this book. But for most breads, especially those that do not have strong structures, it is better to decrease the amount of salt used than to omit it entirely if you are on a low salt diet.

EGGS strengthen the structure of breads and are especially important in gluten-free breads. The recipes in this book call for extra large eggs. If your eggs do not measure ¼ c. each, add a little water to bring them up to ¼ c. volume. Bring the eggs to room temperature and beat them slightly before adding them to your bread. If you forget to take them out of the refrigerator to warm up ahead of baking time, immerse them in a bowl of warm tap water for a few minutes to warm them up quickly.

EGG SUBSTITUTES, such as Egg Beaters™, may be used in place of eggs in the few recipes in this book that call for eggs. By using them, you avoid eating the cholesterol that eggs contain. However, egg substitutes contain eggs whites, and can contain milk or milk derivatives, corn derivatives, and wheat gluten, so they are not a good choice for people with food allergies. They are available refrigerated or frozen, and may be frozen at home.

GUAR GUM is a soluble fiber that comes from a legume. It is used to impart structure to trap the leavening gas in gluten-free and low-gluten breads. Guar gum mixes readily with water, and I feel that it produces a slightly better structure than xanthum gum, but the two can be used interchangeably. Guar gum is more economical than xanthum gum.

XANTHUM GUM is another soluble fiber that can be used to give structure to low-gluten and gluten-free breads. It comes from a bacteria, *Xanthomonas compestris*. It can be substituted for guar gum in the recipes in this book. If your bread comes out very dense, you may wish to increase the amount used by ¼ to ½. Xanthum gum does not mix readily with water, so if you wish to use it, mix it with part of the flour.

VITAMIN C CRYSTALS impart acid to yeast bread dough, which can strengthen the protein structure when used in moderation. It can also be used as the acid leavening component in handmade non-yeast breads. Vitamin C crystals and powder may be used interchangeably. Be sure whatever kind of vitamin C you use is unbuffered, or it will not impart acid to your bread.

RAISINS AND OTHER DRIED FRUITS, NUTS, SEEDS, AND GRAINS OR GRAIN COMPONENTS, such as cracked wheat, cracked spelt, wheat germ, oat bran, and oatmeal are used in some of the recipes in this book to provide extra fiber and a variety of textures and tastes.

Instructions and Recipes For Mixers, Food Processors, & Handmade Quick Breads

If you are not ready to purchase a bread machine, you can still use appliances that you may already have to save yourself time and effort when you make bread. A microwave oven can be used to make your bread rise in a fraction of the time it would normally take. (See pages 18 to 19). An electric mixer can do part, or if it is heavy-duty, all of the work of kneading bread for you, making several loaves at a time. And a food processor can knead your bread in just one minute, although you can knead only one loaf at a time.

Any of the bread machine recipes in this book can also be made by hand or with your mixer. The recipes made with flours that contain a fair amount of gluten, such as wheat, spelt, and kamut, can also be made in a food processor. Breads made by hand or with a mixer or processor may absorb slightly more flour in the kneading process than bread machine breads take, so plan to use a little more flour. Or, especially if you are using your food processor to make the dough, you may prefer to decrease the amount of the water in the bread machine recipe by about ⅛ c. to produce bread of the right consistency, which will be slightly firmer than bread machine bread. Since you can add flour until the "feel" of the dough is right (see page 13), variations in the amount of moisture the flour contains, gluten content, etc. will be compensated for, so accurate measuring is not as critical as with bread machine breads. When making bread by hand or with one of these appliances, the most important factor is how the dough feels when the right amount of flour has been added and the gluten is properly developed. This is something that you will learn with experience.

Instructions are given below for making yeast breads using a food processor or mixer and quick breads by hand. Some sample recipes are also included to guide you as you use the bread machine recipes in the following chapters to make bread by hand, mixer, or processor.

FOOD PROCESSOR BREADS

To make yeast dough in a food processor, put the dough blade or metal blade used for pureeing into the machine. Put the dry ingredients, such as the flour, yeast, salt, dry sweeteners, and spices, in the processor bowl and pulse a few times to mix. Add the oil and lecithin (if you are using it), and pulse a few times until it is absorbed evenly by the flour. Combine the liquid ingredients, such as water and fruit juice, in a cup or bowl. They should be at or slightly above room temperature, about 80°F. Turn the processor on and add the liquid ingredients slowly through the feed tube, reserving about 1 tbsp. of liquid. When the dough forms a ball that cleans the side of the bowl (although there may be a few scraps of dough that do not join the ball), begin timing and process for one minute. Add the last tablespoon of liquid if necessary to make the dough form a ball. If the full amount of liquid does not make the dough form a ball, add an additional tablespoon of water. After the dough has kneaded for one minute, remove it from the processor and knead it briefly by hand on a floured board to check its consistency. If it is too sticky, knead in an additional 1 to 2 tbsp. of flour by hand. This is also the time to add raisins or nuts by hand. Put the dough in an oiled bowl, turn it over, and allow it to rise in a warm (85 to 90°F) place until doubled in volume, about 40 minutes to 1 hour. Or use your microwave oven to proof it as on pages 18 to 19. Punch the dough down and shape it into loaves or rolls as desired. (For loaves, use an 8"x4" or 9"x 5" oiled loaf pan.) Allow it to rise until double again. Bake loaves at 350°F to 375°F, usually for 45 minutes to an hour, and rolls at 375°F for 15 to 25 minutes.

Food Processor White Bread

3⅛ c. bread flour

1¾ tsp. active dry or quick-rise yeast

1 tsp. salt

1 tbsp. oil

½ tbsp. liquid lecithin or additional oil

¼ c. apple juice concentrate at room temperature

¾ c. water at room temperature

Prepare the dough as in the food processor bread directions on page 41, and let it rise once. Punch down the dough and shape it into one loaf. Put it into an oiled loaf pan. Let it rise until it has doubled again, about 45 minutes. Bake at 375°F for 40 to 45 minutes. Immediately remove it from the pan and cool it on a wire rack. Makes 1 loaf. This dough can also be used to make rolls or buns (p. 129 to 141), pizza (p. 180), breadsticks (p. 188), or pretzels (p. 189). The nutritional analysis for this recipe is the same as for a large loaf of "White Bread," p. 61.

Food Processor White Spelt Bread

2⅞ c. white spelt flour

1¾ tsp. active dry or quick-rise yeast

¾ tsp. salt

2½ tsp. oil

1 tsp. liquid lecithin or additional oil

3 tbsp. apple juice concentrate at room temperature

⅝ c. water at room temperature

Prepare the dough as in the food processor bread directions on page 41, and let it rise once. Punch down the dough and shape it into one loaf. Put it into an oiled loaf pan. Let it rise until it has doubled again, about 45 minutes. Bake at 375°F for 40 to 45 minutes. Immediately remove it from the pan and cool it on a wire rack. Makes 1 loaf. This dough can also be used to make rolls or buns (p. 129 to 141), pizza (p. 182), breadsticks (p. 188), or pretzels (p. 189). The nutritional analysis for this recipe is the same as for a large loaf of "White Spelt Bread", p. 63.

Food Processor Whole Wheat Bread

3 c. whole wheat bread flour

1¾ tsp. active dry or quick-rise yeast

¾ tsp. salt

1 tbsp. oil

1 tsp. liquid lecithin or additional oil

3 tbsp. apple juice concentrate at room temperature

1 c. water at room temperature

Prepare the dough as in the food processor bread directions on page 41 and let it rise once. Punch down the dough and shape it into one loaf. Put it into an oiled loaf pan. Let it rise until it has doubled again, about 45 minutes. Bake at 375°F for 40 to 45 minutes. Immediately remove it from the pan and cool it on a wire rack. Makes 1 loaf. This dough can also be used to make rolls or buns (p. 129 to 141), pizza (p. 180), breadsticks (p. 188), or pretzels (p. 189). The nutritional analysis for this recipe is the same as for a small loaf of "100% Whole Wheat Bread," p. 80.

Food Processor Spelt Bread

3⅓ c. whole spelt flour

2¼ tsp. active dry or quick-rise yeast

¾ tsp. salt

1 tbsp. oil

½ tbsp. liquid lecithin or additional oil

¼ c. apple juice concentrate at room temperature

⅞ c. water at room temperature

Prepare the dough as in the food processor bread directions on page 41 and let it rise once. Punch down the dough and shape it into one loaf. Put it into an oiled loaf pan. (This bread is sometimes difficult to remove from the pan after baking, especially if it has been baked for the full baking time. If you prefer your bread well browned, you may want to line the pan with waxed or parchment paper after oiling it and also oil the paper.) Let it rise until it has doubled again, about 45 minutes. Bake at 375°F for 40 to 45 minutes. Immediately run a knife around the edges of the loaf and remove it from the pan. Cool it on a wire rack. Makes 1 loaf. This dough can also be used to make rolls or buns (p. 129 to 141), pita bread (p.125), pizza (p. 182), breadsticks (p. 188), or pretzels (p. 189). The nutritional analysis for this recipe is the same as for a large loaf of "Whole Grain Spelt Bread," p. 91.

Food Processor Kamut Bread

2¼ tsp. active dry or quick-rise yeast

3¼ c. kamut flour

¾ tsp. salt

2 tbsp. oil

¼ c. apple or pineapple juice concentrate
at room temperature

1⅛ c. water at room temperature

Prepare the dough as in the food processor bread directions on page 41 except do not let it rise the first time. After checking its consistency, shape it into a loaf and put it into an oiled loaf pan. Let it rise until it has doubled, about 45 minutes. Bake at 375°F for 40 to 45 minutes. Immediately remove it from the pan and cool it on a wire rack. Makes 1 loaf. This dough can also be used to make rolls or buns (p. 129 to 141), pizza (p. 182), breadsticks (p. 188), or pretzels (p. 189). The nutritional analysis for this recipe is the same as for a small loaf of "Kamut Bread," p. 92.

MIXER BREADS MADE WITH HIGH-GLUTEN FLOURS

To make yeast bread using high-gluten flours, such as wheat, spelt, kamut, or rye, with your mixer, put ½ to ⅔ of the flour, the yeast, the salt, and the other dry ingredients in the mixer bowl. Mix on low speed for about 30 seconds. Warm the liquid ingredients to 115-120°F. With the mixer running on low speed, add the liquids to the dry ingredients in a slow stream. Continue mixing until the dry and liquid ingredients are thoroughly mixed. If your mixer is not a heavy-duty mixer, at this point beat the dough for 5 to 10 minutes. With some types of bread, you will be able to tell that the gluten is developing because the dough will begin to climb up the beaters. Then knead the rest of the flour in by hand, kneading for about 10 minutes, or until the dough is very smooth and elastic. If you wish to add raisins or nuts to the dough, do it during this hand kneading period.

If your mixer is a heavy-duty mixer, after the liquids are thoroughly mixed in, with the mixer still running, begin adding the rest of the flour around the edges of the bowl ½ c. at a time, mixing well after each addition before adding more flour, until the dough forms a ball and cleans the sides of the bowl. Knead the dough on the speed directed in your mixer manual for 5 to 10 minutes, or until the dough is very elastic and smooth. Turn the dough out onto a floured board and knead it briefly to check the consistency of the dough, kneading in a little more flour if necessary. Raisins or nuts should be added to the dough by hand after the mixer is finished kneading it.

Put the dough into an oiled bowl and turn it once so that the top of the ball is also oiled. Cover it with a towel and let it rise in a warm (85°F to 90°F) place until it has doubled in volume, about 45 minutes to 1 hour, or use the microwave rising method on pages 18 to 19. Punch the dough down and shape it into loaves or rolls as desired. (For loaves, use an 8"x 4" or 9"x 5" oiled loaf pan.) Allow it to rise until double again. Bake loaves at 350°F to 375°F, usually for 45 minutes to an hour, and rolls at 375°F for 15 to 25 minutes.

Depending on the capacity of your mixer's bowl and the power of its motor, you can double, triple, or quadruple the recipes given for bread machines and make several loaves of bread at once. The following sample recipes are for two loaves of bread each.

Mixer White Bread

4 c. bread flour

3½ tsp. active dry or quick-rise yeast

2 tsp. salt

½ c. apple juice concentrate warmed to 120°F

1½ c. water at about 120°F

2 tbsp. oil

1 tbsp. liquid lecithin or additional oil

2¼ to 2½ c. bread flour

Prepare the dough as in the mixer bread directions on pages 44 to 45. After the first rise, punch down the dough and shape it into two loaves. Put each loaf into an oiled loaf pan. Let the loaves rise until they have doubled again, about 45 minutes. Bake at 375°F for 40 to 45 minutes. Immediately remove the bread from the pans and cool it on a wire rack. Makes 2 loaves. This recipe may be doubled if your mixer is capable of kneading four loaves of bread. The dough from this recipe can also be used to make rolls or buns (p. 129 to 141), pizza (p. 180), breadsticks (p. 188), or pretzels (p. 189). The nutritional analysis for this bread is the same as for two large loaves of "White Bread," page 61.

Mixer White Spelt Bread

4 c. white spelt flour

3½ tsp. active dry or quick-rise yeast

1½ tsp. salt

⅜ c. apple juice concentrate warmed to 120°F

1¼ c. water at about 120°F

5 tsp. oil

2 tsp. liquid lecithin or additional oil

1¾ to 2 c. white spelt flour

Prepare the dough as in the mixer bread directions on pages 44 to 45. After the first rise, punch down the dough and shape it into two loaves. Put each loaf into an oiled loaf pan. Let the loaves rise until they have doubled again, about 45 minutes. Bake at 375°F for 40 to 45 minutes. Immediately remove the bread from the pans and cool it on a wire rack. Makes 2 loaves. This recipe may be doubled if your mixer is capable of kneading four loaves of bread. The dough from this recipe can also be used to make rolls or buns (p. 129 to 141), pizza (p. 182), breadsticks (p. 188), or pretzels (p. 189). The nutritional analysis for this bread is the same as for two large loaves of "White Spelt Bread," page 63.

Mixer Whole Wheat Bread

4½ c. whole wheat bread flour

2 packages (4½ tsp.) active dry or quick-rise yeast

2 tsp. salt

½ c. apple juice concentrate warmed to 120°F

2¼ c. water at about 120°F

2 tbsp. oil

1 tbsp. liquid lecithin or additional oil

3 to 3 ¼ c. whole wheat bread flour

Prepare the dough as in the mixer bread directions on pages 44 to 45. After the first rise, punch down the dough and shape it into two loaves. Put each loaf into an oiled loaf pan. Let the loaves rise until they have doubled again, about 45 minutes. Bake at 375°F for 40 to 45 minutes. Immediately remove the bread from the pans and cool it on a wire rack. Makes 2 loaves. This recipe may be doubled if your mixer is capable of kneading four loaves of bread. The dough from this recipe can also be used to make rolls or buns (p. 129 to 141), pizza (p. 180), breadsticks (p. 188), or pretzels (p. 189). The nutritional analysis for this bread is the same as for two large loaves of "100% Whole Wheat Bread," page 80.

Mixer Spelt Bread

> 4 c. spelt flour
>
> 2 packages (4½ tsp.) active dry or quick-rise yeast
>
> 1¼ tsp. salt
>
> ⅓ c. apple juice concentrate warmed to 120°F
>
> 1⅔ c. water at about 120°F
>
> 2 tbsp. oil
>
> 1 tbsp. liquid lecithin or additional oil
>
> 2¼ to 2¾ c. spelt flour

Prepare the dough as in the mixer bread directions on pages 44 to 45. After the first rise, punch down the dough and shape it into two loaves. Put each loaf into an oiled loaf pan. (This bread is sometimes difficult to remove from the pan after baking, especially if it has been baked for the full baking time. If you prefer your bread well browned, you may want to line the pans with parchment paper or waxed paper after oiling them and also oil the paper.) Let the loaves rise until they have doubled again, about 45 minutes. Bake at 375°F for 40 to 45 minutes. Immediately run a knife around the edges of the loaves and remove them from the pans. Cool them on a wire rack. Makes 2 loaves. This recipe may be doubled if your mixer is capable of kneading four loaves of bread. The dough from this recipe can also be used to make rolls or buns (p. 129 to 141), pizza (p. 182), breadsticks (p. 188), or pretzels (p. 189). The nutritional analysis for this bread is the same as for two large loaves of "Whole Grain Spelt Bread," page 91.

Mixer Kamut Bread

> 4 c. kamut flour
>
> 2 packages (4½ tsp.) active dry or quick-rise yeast
>
> 1½ tsp. salt
>
> 2½ c. water at about 120°F
>
> ½ c. apple or pineapple juice concentrate
>   warmed to 120°F
>
> 3 tbsp. oil
>
> 2½ to 3 c. kamut flour

Prepare the dough as in the mixer bread directions on pages 44 to 45, except do not let it rise the first time. After checking the consistency of the dough, shape the dough into two loaves. Put each loaf into an oiled 8″ by 4″ loaf pan. Let the loaves rise in a warm place until they double or reach the top of the pans, about 30 to 50 minutes. Bake at 375°F for 40 to 45 minutes. Remove the loaves from the pans immediately. Cool them on a wire rack. Makes 2 loaves. This recipe may be doubled if your mixer is capable of kneading four loaves of bread. The dough from this recipe can be used in rolls or buns (p. 129 to 141), pizza (p. 182), breadsticks (p. 188), or pretzels (p. 189). The nutritional analysis for this bread is the same as for two small loaves of "Kamut Bread," p. 92.

Mixer Brown Bread

4 c. white rye flour (see "Sources," p. 236)
3 packages (6¾ tbsp.) active dry or quick-rise yeast
1 tbsp. salt
2 tbsp. caraway seeds
¼ c. carob (optional - if omitted, add an
    extra ¼. c. flour)
2 c. water at about 120°F
½ c. dark molasses
2 tbsp. oil
3¼ to 3¾ c. white rye flour

Prepare the dough as in the mixer bread directions on pages 44 to 45. After the first rise, punch down the dough and shape it into two balls. Place them on oiled baking sheets and slash the tops of the loaves. Let them rise until double in volume, about one hour. Bake at 375°F for 35 to 45 minutes. Makes two loaves. The nutritional analysis for this bread is the same as for two loaves of "Brown Bread," p. 89.

MIXER BREADS MADE WITH GLUTEN-FREE AND LOW-GLUTEN FLOURS

Gluten-free and low-gluten breads are much different than high-gluten breads. Instead of your mixer developing the gluten, it "develops" the guar gum structure of the bread. Because low-gluten and gluten-free bread dough is much softer, ranging in consistency from a heavy batter to a soft dough, all of the "kneading" can be done by your mixer even if it is not a heavy duty mixer. The beating times are shorter (about 3 minutes) for gluten-free and low-gluten breads than for gluten-containing mixer breads. Also, you beat the dough twice, once initially and once after the first rising period. The method described in the two sample recipes below can also be used to make barley, oat, amaranth, quinoa, and buckwheat breads and gluten-free rolls or sweet rolls. (See the bread machine recipes on pages 93 to 98, 128, 140, and 222.) Use the same amounts of all of the ingredients as in the bread machine recipes. The rising and baking times will vary with the type of bread you make. Just let the bread rise until it barely doubles and bake it until it is brown. DO NOT let these breads over-rise in the pan or they will collapse during baking.

Mixer Rice Bread

    2 c. brown rice flour or white rice flour

    ⅓ c. potato flour

    ⅓ c. tapioca flour

    1 package (2¼ tsp.) active dry or quick-rise yeast

    4 tsp. guar gum

    ⅛ tsp. unbuffered vitamin C crystals

    1 tsp. salt

    2 tbsp. oil

    3 extra-large eggs OR ¾ c. egg substitute
      at room temperature

    ¼ c. apple juice concentrate at about 115°F

    ½ c. water at about 115°F

Combine the flours, yeast, guar gum, vitamin C crystals, and salt in your large mixer bowl and mix for about 30 seconds. Beat the eggs slightly and combine them with the water, juice, and oil in a separate bowl or cup. With the mixer running, add the liquid ingredients to the bowl. When the ingredients are completely combined, beat the dough for three minutes at medium speed. Scrape the dough from the beaters and the sides of the bowl into the bottom of the bowl. Cover the bowl, put it in a warm (85°F to 90°F) place, and let the dough rise for 1 hour. Beat the dough again for three minutes at medium speed. Oil an 8" by 4" loaf pan and coat the inside of it generously with rice flour. Put the dough in the pan and allow it to rise in a warm place until it doubles, about 30 to 40 minutes for active dry yeast or 20 to 30 minutes for quick-rise yeast. Preheat the oven to 375°F. Bake for 30 to 45 minutes. Makes one loaf. The nutritional analysis of this recipe is the same as for a large loaf of "Gluten-free Rice Potato Bread," p. 76.

Mixer Egg-free Rice Bread

2¾ c. brown rice flour

¾ c. tapioca flour

1 package (2¼ tsp.) active dry or quick-rise yeast

1 tbsp. guar gum

1 tsp. salt

1½ c. warm (110-115°F) water

3 tbsp. honey or Fruit Sweet™

3 tbsp. oil

Combine the flours, yeast, guar gum, and salt in your large mixer bowl and mix for about 30 seconds. Combine the water, honey or Fruit Sweet™, and oil in a separate bowl or cup. With the mixer running, add the liquid ingredients to the bowl. When the ingredients are completely combined, beat the dough for three minutes at medium speed. Scrape the dough from the beaters and the sides of the bowl into the bottom of the bowl. Cover the bowl, put it in a warm (85°F to 90°F) place, and let the dough rise for 1 hour. Beat the dough again for three minutes at medium speed. Oil an 8" by 4" or 9" by 5" loaf pan and coat the inside of it generously with rice flour. Put the dough in the pan and allow it to rise in a warm place until it doubles, about 25 to 35 minutes for active dry yeast or 20 to 25 minutes for quick-rise yeast. Preheat the

oven to 375°F. Bake for 30 to 45 minutes. Makes one loaf.
The nutritional analysis of this recipe is the same as for
"Egg-free Brown Rice Bread," p. 96.

HAND MIXED QUICK BREADS

Quick breads are very easy to make by hand without
any machines. (But if you are on a yeast-free diet and eat quick
breads exclusively, it is nice to have a bread machine that will do
the work for you!) To make quick breads by hand, first preheat
your oven to 350°F and oil and flour your bread pan. Stir
together the flour(s), baking powder, baking soda, salt, and
other dry ingredients in a large bowl. Combine the liquid ingredients in another bowl or cup. Stir them into the dry ingredients quickly, until they are just barely mixed together, and put
the batter into the prepared pan. Bake at 350°F until the bread
is nicely browned and a toothpick inserted in the center comes
out dry. This may take from 30 to 70 minutes. When adapting
the bread machine quick bread recipes in this book, there is no
need to change the amounts of any of the ingredients. Some
sample hand mixed quick bread recipes are given on the next
two pages.

Hand Mixed Corn Bread

> 1½ c. all purpose flour
>
> ½ c. cornmeal
>
> 2½ tsp. baking powder
>
> ½ tsp. salt
>
> 2 tbsp. oil
>
> 1 extra large egg OR ¼ c. egg substitute
>   OR ¼ c. water in addition to the amount below
>
> ¼ c. Fruit Sweet™ or honey
>
> ⅜ c. water

Preheat your oven to 350°F. Oil and flour an 8″ by 4″ loaf pan. Mix together the flour, cornmeal, baking powder, and salt in a large bowl. Combine the oil, egg, sweetener, and water and quickly stir them into the dry ingredients until they are just mixed. Put the batter into the prepared pan and bake at 350°F for 30 to 40 minutes, or until the bread is golden brown and a toothpick inserted into the center comes out clean. The nutritional analysis for this bread is the same as for "Corn Bread," p. 153.

Hand Mixed White Spelt Quick Bread

> 3 c. white spelt flour
>
> 3 tsp. baking powder
>
> ½ tsp. salt
>
> ¼ c. oil
>
> 1 c. water

Preheat your oven to 350°F. Oil and flour (with white spelt flour) an 8″ by 4″ loaf pan. Mix together the flour, baking powder, and salt in a large bowl. Combine the oil and water and quickly stir them into the dry ingredients until they are just mixed. Put the batter into the prepared pan and bake at 350°F for 60 to 70 minutes, or until the bread is golden brown and a toothpick inserted into the center comes out clean. This bread is fragile, so allow it to cool completely before slicing it. The nutritional analysis for this bread is the same as for "No-Yeast White Spelt Bread", p. 145.

Hand Mixed
White Rice Quick Bread

1⅓ c. white rice flour

⅓ c. tapioca flour

⅓ c. potato flour

2¾ tsp. guar gum

2¾ tsp. baking powder

¾ tsp. salt

1 tbsp. plus 1 tsp. oil

2 extra-large eggs, slightly beaten,
   OR ½ c. egg substitute

1⅓ c. water

Preheat your oven to 350°F. Oil and flour (with white rice flour) an 8″ by 4″ loaf pan. Mix together the flours, baking powder, guar gum, and salt in a large bowl. Combine the oil, eggs, and water and quickly stir them into the dry ingredients until they are just mixed. Put the batter into the prepared pan and bake at 350°F for 55 to 65 minutes, or until the bread is golden brown and a toothpick inserted into the center comes out clean. The nutritional analysis for this bread is the same as for "No-Yeast Gluten-free Rice Bread," p. 152.

Instructions & Recipes for Bread Machine Breads

Each bread machine has a personality of its own (at our house, they even have names), so the first thing you should do when you get a bread machine is get to know it. Read the instruction booklet and any recipes that come with it. Make a basic bread with a recipe the manufacturer provides. Listen to how the machine sounds as it kneads. Reach into the machine and feel the dough. If the times for each part of the cycle are not given in the instruction book, time the parts of the cycle. Peek into the machine and see how the dough looks at every stage of the cycle.

Getting to know your bread machine is helpful in many ways. When you know how it normally sounds, you will recognize the distressed kneading sound it makes if your dough is too stiff and dry. If you know how long each part of the cycle takes, you will know when the last knead ends and can set your kitchen timer to add raisins or nuts near the end of the kneading time. Touching the dough will give you experience in how bread machine dough should feel.

An important skill to develop is the ability to judge the consistency of the dough by looking at it and touching it. For high-gluten doughs, such as wheat and spelt, after several minutes of kneading, the dough should form a smooth, silky ball. It should feel slightly tacky, but not sticky, when you reach into the machine and touch it. Do not judge a bread dough and begin adding flour or water in the first few minutes of kneading; allow the gluten time to develop. (The exception to this is if the machine sounds like it is really laboring to knead. In this case, add water 1 tbsp. at a time immediately.) After several minutes of kneading, if the dough is too wet or too dry, add either flour (1 tbsp. at a time) or water (1 tsp. at a time) until the right consistency is reached, allowing the machine to knead for a minute or two after each addition. Using this method, you can compensate for the inevitable variations in flour quality or moisture content due to weather changes.

Record any changes you make in the recipes and how they turn out. If you live in an exceptionally dry or wet climate, you may find that you routinely have to use more water or flour than the recipe calls for.

The consistency of lower-gluten doughs varies from recipe to recipe and is difficult to make generalizations about. Rye doughs are very sticky. Some gluten-free doughs may look and feel more like heavy batters than doughs. The first time you make each unusual bread, follow the recipe exactly and observe the consistency of the dough carefully. Measuring accurately and using high quality ingredients should produce a good loaf, but if your bread does not come out well, record that, and make the appropriate changes (see below) the next time, again observing the dough. After making a few loaves of each kind of bread, you will gain enough experience to be able to compensate for any variations in your flour easily. Using high quality commercial flours the first few times you make these types of bread is highly recommended.

The most common problem you will have making non-wheat bread is that the loaf will collapse during baking. This collapse may be very slight, just resulting in a flat-topped loaf, and may not even need correcting. Or the collapse can be profound and the loaf can come out with a sunken top or gooey in the middle. There are several possible causes and solutions for this problem. One possible cause is that the dough may have been too wet. Increase the amount of flour or decrease the amount of water the next time you make the bread. Another cause may be that the second rising time is too long. If you have a programmable machine, decrease the last rising time. To slow the rising, you may also decrease the amount of yeast or slightly increase the amount of salt used. You can also try to increase the structure strength of the bread by increasing the amount of guar gum you use. Or, if you are not allergic to eggs, you can strengthen the bread's structure by replacing part of the water called for with eggs, using one extra large egg instead of ¼ c. of water.

It is very important to measure accurately when using a bread machine. To measure flour, stir it to loosen it, lightly spoon it into your measuring cup, and level it off with a straight-edged knife or spatula. To measure liquids, place the measuring cup on a flat surface, and get down so your eye is at the level of the cup to read it. The bottom of the curve of the liquid (meniscus) should line up with the measurement you want to use. When measuring dry ingredients in a measuring spoon, level them off with a straight-edged knife or spatula. When measuring liquids, make sure they do not round up above the top of the spoon.

All ingredients should be at or slightly above room temperature when they go into the bread machine. Eggs can be warmed up quickly by immersing them in warm tap water for a few minutes. Microwave ovens are great for bringing other cold ingredients up to room temperature; just be careful not to microwave them for too long.

Add the ingredients to the pan in the order that the manufacturer of your bread machine recommends. This will either be from the top down or from the bottom up as you read the recipe. Occasionally I have reversed the order by mistake. When I have added the yeast first to a liquids-first machine, the machine had difficulty mixing the dough. But when I added the liquids first to a yeast-first machine there were no problems. When you are using the delayed cycle timer, it is better to add the liquids first and put the yeast in a small well in the top of the flour to insure that it stays dry, even if you normally add the yeast first. The ingredients are listed in a specific order in each recipe to keep the yeast from coming into contact with the salt, oil, or liquids during any waiting time before the machine mixes the dough.

Most of the time, bread machines do not need any attention after you start them, but if you are going to be nearby when they are running, it is worth your while to peek into them a couple of times during the cycle. If you check the dough's consistency after the first several minutes of mixing, you will know if you forgot to put in a cup of the flour or if the weather has made a little adjustment necessary, and can correct the problem early to insure a good loaf of bread. Also, if you look into the machine during the rising time, you will be able to puncture the dough with a pin if it is threatening to rise over the edge of the pan. (This should only occur if you are "experimenting.") Also, you will know if you have forgotten to add the yeast. I have occasionally added yeast to the pan at this point, started the cycle over again, and had good results.

For some machines and some recipes, such as the Zojirushi BBCC-S15 with some non-wheat breads, the machine will be unable to mix in all of the flour if it is added to the pan at the beginning of the cycle. Reserve about ⅓ of the flour and add it to the machine after the first part is well mixed in by sprinkling it around the outer edges of the pan ¼ c. at a time.

When you make bread with some of the unusual non-wheat flours, the machine will require some assistance in mixing the batter or dough. For the Welbilt ABM-150R machine, with its round pan and powerful motor, this consists in using a rubber spatula to detach the dough from the sides of the pan and possibly pushing the upper central part of the dough to the side so it will be thoroughly mixed in. For other machines, especially those with square pans, you may also need use the rubber spatula to carefully turn the dough over in the pan. In the Welbilt machine, you can forget to assist with mixing the dough in some recipes that call for it, and the bread will still come out fine. Most bread machine instruction booklets caution against inserting any utensils into the machine while it is running, but to make many non-wheat breads, careful assistance with a rubber spatula during mixing is a necessity. Also, for some recipes, it is helpful to spread the dough or batter evenly in the pan after the last kneading before the final rise and bake parts of the cycle.

All of the recipes in this book were baked on a medium crust darkness setting. If your machine has a crust color selection feature, the first time you make each recipe, use the medium setting. Then if you prefer your crust darker or lighter, make a note of it and try a different setting the next time.

The recipes in this book give the amounts of ingredients to use to make 1 lb. or 1½ lb. loaves. If your machine can make 2 lb. loaves, first try making a 1½ lb. loaf to see if it almost fills the pan. If is does, a 2 lb. loaf will probably be a "lid thumper." If not, you can make a 2 lb. loaf by doubling the amounts of the ingredients given for a 1 lb. loaf. If the loaf is very large, decrease the yeast by ¼ tsp. to ½ tsp. the next time.

WHAT TO DO IF...

If you find that your bread is not as light and fluffy as you desire, you may try increasing the amount of the yeast slightly. Some experienced bakers routinely use about 3 tsp. yeast for each 1½ lb. loaf of bread because they prefer very light bread. This may lead to over-rising and collapse with some non-wheat breads, however.

If you live at a very high altitude (over 7000 feet) and your bread over-proofs and collapses during baking, try decreasing the amount of yeast called for in the recipe by ¼ to ⅓.

If you live in a very humid or very dry climate, or if you are baking on an exceptionally dry or rainy day, you may need to compensate for the humidity, or lack of it, when you make bread. Check the dough after several minutes of kneading (see p. 55) and add extra water 1 tsp. at a time or extra flour 1 tbsp. at a time if necessary.

If you already have a non-programmable machine and want to make breads that require a programmable cycle, you can use the dough cycle of your machine to make the dough and allow it to rise the first time. Then transfer the dough to an oiled loaf pan, allow it to rise until barely doubled, and bake it in the oven at 350°F until it is nicely browned. For very dense breads, this may take over an hour.

If your machine does not have a whole grain cycle and your whole grain breads come out very dense, they may benefit from some extra kneading time. Simply stop the machine and start the cycle over again after the first 15 to 20 minutes of kneading and then let the cycle proceed normally.

If your machine has a rectangular pan and you notice that there are floury patches on the corners of the finished loaf of bread, the next time you bake, check the bread after it has kneaded for several minutes. If there is still flour in the corners of the pan, use a rubber spatula to move it so it will be kneaded into the dough.

If your bread does not rise at all, think back. Did you remember to put the yeast into the machine? One of the advantages of machines that specify adding the yeast first and liquids last is that it is much harder to forget to add the yeast! But if there are children at your house, they love to play with inedible loaves of bread.

If you have other problems, you may wish to call your bread machine manufacturer for advice. Also, Red Star Yeast has a bread machine information line. Along with answering your questions, they may send you coupons to use the next time you purchase yeast. The Red Star Yeast line phone number is 800-445-4746.

Basic Breads

White Bread

Ingredients:	1½ lb. loaf	1 lb. loaf
Water or milk	1 c.	⅔ c.
Fruit Sweet™ or honey	2 tbsp.	4 tsp.
Oil	1 tbsp.	2 tsp.
Liquid lecithin (or may use additional oil)	½ tbsp.	1 tsp.
Salt	1 tsp.	¾ tsp.
Bread flour	3 c.	2 c.
Active dry yeast	1¾ tsp.	1¼ tsp.

Cycle: Basic yeast bread

Nutritional Analysis: (% Daily Value based on a 2000 calorie diet)

	Large Loaf	Small Loaf	Per serving	%D.V.
Calories:	1557	1168	82	4%
Protein (g):	43	32	2.3	-
Carbohydrate (g):	286	214	15	5%
Total fat (g):	23	17	1.2	2%
Saturated (g):	0	0	0	0
Cholesterol (mg):	0	0	0	0
Sodium (mg):	2031	1523	107	4%
Fiber (g):	0.9	0.7	0.05	<1%

Serving size: approximately 1.2 oz.
Servings per large loaf: 19
Servings per small loaf: 14

Diabetic exchanges per serving: 1 starch/bread
Diabetic exchanges per large loaf recipe: 19 starch/bread

No-Salt-Added White Bread

Ingredients:	1½ lb. loaf	1 lb. loaf
Water	⅔ c.	⅜ c. + 1 tbsp.
Apple juice concentrate, thawed	3 tbsp.	2 tbsp.
Oil	2 tsp.	1½ tsp.
Liquid lecithin (or may use additional oil)	1 tsp.	1 tsp.
Bread flour	2⅛c. + 1 tbsp.	1½ c. +1 tbsp.
Active dry yeast	1¼ tsp.	¾ tsp.

Cycle: Basic yeast bread

Nutritional Analysis: (% Daily Value based on a 2000 calorie diet)

	Large Loaf	Small Loaf	Per serving	%D.V.
Calories:	1188	779	79	4%
Protein (g):	32	22	2	-
Carbohydrate (g):	214	143	14.3	5%
Total fat (g):	17	11	1	2%
Saturated (g):	0	0	0	0
Cholesterol (mg):	0	0	0	0
Sodium (mg):	23	15	1.5	<1%
Fiber (g):	0.7	0.5	0.05	<1%

Serving size: approximately 1.0 oz.
Servings per large loaf: 15
Servings per small loaf: 10

Diabetic exchanges per serving: 1 starch/bread
Diabetic exchanges per large loaf recipe: 15 starch/bread

White Spelt Bread

Ingredients:	1½ lb. loaf	1 lb. loaf
Water	¾ c.	⅔ c.
Apple juice concentrate, thawed	3 tbsp.	2 tbsp.
Oil	2½ tsp.	2 tsp.
Liquid lecithin (or may use additional oil)	1 tsp.	1 tsp.
Salt	¾ tsp.	½ tsp.
White spelt flour	2⅞ c.	2⅜ c.
Active dry yeast	1¾ tsp.	1¼ tsp.

Cycle: Basic yeast bread

Nutritional Analysis: (% Daily Value based on a 2000 calorie diet)

	Large Loaf	Small Loaf	Per serving	%D.V.
Calories:	1432	1189	80	4%
Protein (g):	48	40	3	-
Carbohydrate (g):	265	220	15	5%
Total fat (g):	21	17	1.2	2%
Saturated (g):	0	0	0	0
Cholesterol (mg):	0	0	0	0
Sodium (mg):	1526	1267	85	4
Fiber (g):	6	5	0.3	1%

Serving size: approximately 1.0 oz.
Servings per large loaf: 18
Servings per small loaf: 15

Diabetic exchanges per serving: 1 starch/bread
Diabetic exchanges per large loaf recipe: 18 starch/bread

No-Salt-Added White Spelt Bread

Ingredients:	1½ lb. programmable machine
Water	⅔ c.
Apple juice concentrate, thawed	2 tbsp. + 2 tsp.
Oil	2 tsp.
Liquid lecithin (or may use additional oil)	1 tsp.
White spelt flour	2½ c.
Active dry yeast	1½ tsp.

Cycle: Welbilt AMB-150R Multi-logic cycle - Knead 2 = 20 minutes, Rise 2 =35 minutes, Bake = 50 minutes

Cycle: Zojirushi BBCC-S15 - Knead 1 = 10 minutes, Rest = 5 minutes, Knead 2 = 20 minutes, Rise 1 = 5 minutes, Rise 2 = 35 minutes, Bake = 50 minutes

If you do not have a programmable machine, the basic yeast cycle, or if you have it, a quick yeast cycle may be used for this recipe. However, because the gluten structure of white spelt is fragile without salt, the bread may be somewhat coarse in textured and may collapse slightly during baking.

Nutritional Analysis: (% Daily Value based on a 2000 calorie diet)

	Per Loaf	Per serving	%D.V.
Calories:	1245	83	4%
Protein (g):	42	3	-
Carbohydrate (g):	231	15	5%
Total fat (g):	18	1.2	2%
Saturated (g):	0	0	0
Cholesterol (mg):	0	0	0
Sodium (mg):	26	1.7	<1%
Fiber (g):	5	0.3	1%

Serving size: approximately 1.0 oz.; Servings per loaf: 15
Diabetic exchanges per serving: 1 starch/bread
Diabetic exchanges per large loaf recipe: 15 starch/bread

Italian Bread

Ingredients: **1½ lb. or 1 lb. machine**

Water 1¼ c.

Apple juice concentrate, thawed 1½ tbsp.

Salt 1½ tsp.

Bread flour 3¼ c.

Active dry yeast 2¼ tsp.

Cycle: Dough cycle. Remove the dough from the machine at the end of the cycle and knead it briefly on an oiled or very lightly floured board. Shape it into a long or round loaf, or divide it into three pieces, roll them into 15″ ropes, and braid the dough. Place the loaf on a baking sheet that has been oiled and sprinkled with cornmeal. Let it rise in a warm place until double, 30 to 45 minutes. Preheat your oven to 400°F and, if desired, put in a few potatoes to bake along with the bread for added moisture to help the crust become crisp. Spray the bread with water right before baking. Bake for 25 to 40 minutes, spraying it with water twice more after 5 and 10 minutes of baking.

Nutritional Analysis: (% Daily Value based on a 2000 calorie diet)

	Per Loaf	Per serving	%D.V.
Calories:	1362	76	4%
Protein (g):	45	3	-
Carbohydrate (g):	279	15	5%
Total fat (g):	3.6	0.2	<1%
Saturated (g):	0	0	0
Cholesterol (mg):	0	0	0
Sodium (mg):	3022	168	7%
Fiber (g):	1	0.06	<1%

Serving size: approximately 1.3 oz.; Servings per loaf: 18

Diabetic exchanges per serving: 1 starch/bread
Diabetic exchanges per recipe: 18 starch/bread

Wheat-free Italian Bread

Ingredients:	1½ lb. or 1 lb. machine
Water	1¼ c.
Apple juice concentrate, thawed	1½ tbsp.
Salt	1½ tsp.
White spelt flour	3¾ c.
Active dry yeast	2¼ tsp.

Cycle: Dough cycle. Remove the dough from the machine at the end of the cycle and knead it briefly on an oiled or very lightly floured board. Shape it into a long or round loaf, or divide it into three pieces, roll them into 15″ ropes, and braid the dough. Place the loaf on a baking sheet that has been oiled and sprinkled with cornmeal or white spelt flour. Let it rise in a warm place until double, 30 to 45 minutes. Preheat your oven to 400°F and, if desired, put in a few potatoes to bake along with the bread for added moisture to help the crust become crisp. Spray the bread with water right before baking. Bake for 25 to 40 minutes, spraying it with water twice more after 5 and 10 minutes of baking.

Nutritional Analysis: (% Daily Value based on a 2000 calorie diet)

	Per Loaf	Per serving	%D.V.
Calories:	1618	81	4%
Protein (g):	63	3	-
Carbohydrate (g):	328	16	6%
Total fat (g):	7	0.4	<1%
Saturated (g):	0	0	0
Cholesterol (mg):	0	0	0
Sodium (mg):	3022	151	6%
Fiber (g):	7.5	0.4	1%

Serving size: approximately 1.15 oz.; Servings per loaf: 20

Diabetic exchanges per serving: 1 starch/bread
Diabetic exchanges per recipe: 20 starch/bread

French Bread

Ingredients:	1½ lb. or 1 lb. machine
Water	1¼ c.
Apple juice concentrate, thawed	1½ tbsp.
Salt	1½ tsp.
Bread flour	3¼ c.
Active dry yeast	2¼ tsp.

½ slightly beaten egg white OR "Bread or Bun Wash," p. 129

Cycle: Dough cycle, using the ingredients above the dotted line. Remove the dough from the machine at the end of the cycle and knead it briefly on an oiled or very lightly floured board. Shape it into a long loaf or two very thin long loaves. Put it into oiled french bread or baguette pans or on a baking sheet that has been oiled and sprinkled with cornmeal. Brush with egg white or bread wash, slash the top diagonally, and let it rise in a warm place until double, about 30 to 45 minutes. If desired, brush again right before baking. Preheat your oven to 400°F and, if desired, put in a few potatoes to bake along with the bread for added moisture to help the crust become crisp. Bake for 20 to 40 minutes, or until nicely browned.

Nutritional Analysis: (% Daily Value based on a 2000 calorie diet)

	Per Loaf	Per serving	%D.V.
Calories:	1378	77	4%
Protein (g):	49	3	-
Carbohydrate (g):	279	15	5%
Total fat (g):	3.6	0.2	<1%
Saturated (g):	0	0	0
Cholesterol (mg):	0	0	0
Sodium (mg):	3022	168	7%
Fiber (g):	1	0.06	<1%

Serving size: approximately 1.3 oz.; Servings per loaf: 18
Diabetic exchanges per serving: 1 starch/bread
Diabetic exchanges per recipe: 18 starch/bread

Wheat-free French Bread

Ingredients:	1½ lb. or 1 lb. machine
Water	1¼ c.
Apple juice concentrate, thawed	1½ tbsp.
Salt	1½ tsp.
White spelt flour	3¾ c.
Active dry yeast	2¼ tsp.

½ slightly beaten egg white OR "Bread or Bun Wash," p. 129

Cycle: Dough cycle, using the ingredients above the dotted line. Remove the dough from the machine at the end of the cycle and knead it briefly on an oiled or very lightly floured board. Shape it into a long loaf or two very thin long loaves. Put it into oiled french bread or baguette pans or on a baking sheet that has been oiled and sprinkled with cornmeal or white spelt flour. Brush with egg white or bread wash, slash the top diagonally, and let it rise in a warm place until double, about 30 to 45 minutes. If desired, brush again right before baking. Preheat your oven to 400°F and, if desired, put in a few potatoes to bake along with the bread for added moisture to help the crust become crisp. Bake for 20 to 40 minutes, or until nicely browned.

Nutritional Analysis: (% Daily Value based on a 2000 calorie diet)

	Per Loaf	Per serving	%D.V.
Calories:	1634	82	4%
Protein (g):	67	3	-
Carbohydrate (g):	328	16	6%
Total fat (g):	7	0.4	<1%
Saturated (g):	0	0	0
Cholesterol (mg):	0	0	0
Sodium (mg):	3022	15	6%
Fiber (g):	7.5	0.4	1%

Serving size: approximately 1.15 oz.; Servings per loaf: 20
Diabetic exchanges per serving: 1 starch/bread
Diabetic exchanges per recipe: 20 starch/bread

Oat Bran Bread

Ingredients:	1½ lb. loaf	1 lb. loaf
Water	1 c.	¾ c.
Apple juice concentrate, thawed	¼ c.	3 tbsp.
Oil	2 tsp.	1½ tsp.
Liquid lecithin (or may use additional oil)	1 tsp.	½ tsp.
Salt	1 tsp.	¾ tsp.
Bread flour	2⅔ c.	2 c.
Oat bran	¾ c.	½ c. + 1 tbsp.
Active dry yeast	1¾ tsp.	1¼ tsp.

Cycle: Basic yeast bread

Nutritional Analysis: (% Daily Value based on a 2000 calorie diet)

	Large Loaf	Small Loaf	Per serving	%D.V.
Calories:	1509	1132	84	4%
Protein (g):	46	35	2.6	-
Carbohydrate (g):	269	202	15	5%
Total fat (g):	26	20	1.4	2%
Saturated (g):	0	0	0	0
Cholesterol (mg):	0	0	0	0
Sodium (mg):	2039	1529	113	5%
Fiber (g):	9	7	0.3	1%

Serving size: approximately 1.25 oz.
Servings per large loaf: 18
Servings per small loaf: 14

Diabetic exchanges per serving: 1 starch/bread
Diabetic exchanges per large loaf recipe: 18 starch/bread

No-Salt-Added Oat Bran Bread

Ingredients:	1½ lb. loaf	1 lb. loaf
Water	¾ c.	⅝ c.
Apple juice concentrate, thawed	3 tbsp.	2 tbsp. + ¾ tsp.
Oil	2 tsp.	1 tsp.
Liquid lecithin (or may use additional oil)	1 tsp.	1 tsp.
Bread flour	2 c.	1½ c.
Oat bran	½ c. + 1 tbsp.	⅜ c. + 2 tsp.
Active dry yeast	1¼ tsp.	¾ tsp.

Cycle: Basic yeast bread

Nutritional Analysis: (% Daily Value based on a 2000 calorie diet)

	Large Loaf	Small Loaf	Per serving	%D.V.
Calories:	1116	837	80	4%
Protein (g):	35	26	2.5	-
Carbohydrate (g):	201	151	14	5%
Total fat (g):	18	13	1.3	2%
Saturated (g):	0	0	0	0
Cholesterol (mg):	0	0	0	0
Sodium (mg):	32	24	2.3	<1%
Fiber (g):	7	5	0.8	3%

Serving size: approximately 1.2 oz.
Servings per large loaf: 14;   Servings per small loaf: 11

Diabetic exchanges per serving: 1 starch/bread
Diabetic exchanges per large loaf recipe: 14 starch/bread

Wheat-free Oat Bran Bread

Ingredients:	1½ lb. loaf	1 lb. loaf
Water	1 c.	¾ c. + 1 tbsp.
Apple juice concentrate, thawed	¼ c.	3 tbsp.
Oil	1 tbsp.	2 tsp.
Liquid lecithin (or may use additional oil)	½ tbsp.	1 tsp.
Salt	¾ tsp.	½ tsp.
White spelt flour	3 c.	2⅓ c.
Oat bran	¾ c.	½ c. + 1 tbsp.
Active dry yeast	2¼ tsp.	1½ tsp.

Cycle: Basic yeast bread

Nutritional Analysis: (% Daily Value based on a 2000 calorie diet)

	Large Loaf	Small Loaf	Per serving	%D.V.
Calories:	1691	1268	85	4%
Protein (g):	60	45	3	-
Carbohydrate (g):	303	227	15	5%
Total fat (g):	29	22	1.4	2%
Saturated (g):	0	0	0	0
Cholesterol (mg):	0	0	0	0
Sodium (mg):	1539	1154	77	3%
Fiber (g):	14	10.5	0.7	3%

Serving size: approximately 1.15 oz.
Servings per large loaf: 20
Servings per small loaf: 16

Diabetic exchanges per serving: 1 starch/bread
Diabetic exchanges per large loaf recipe: 20 starch/bread

Oatmeal Bread

Ingredients:	1½ lb. loaf	1 lb. loaf
Boiling water	1 c.	¾ c.
Uncooked rolled oats or quick rolled oats	½ c.	⅜ c.
Apple juice concentrate, thawed	¼ c.	3 tbsp.
Oil	1 tbsp.	2 tsp.
Liquid lecithin (or may use additional oil)	½ tbsp.	1 tsp.
Salt	1 tsp.	¾ tsp.
Bread flour	2⅝ c.	2 c.
Active dry yeast	1¾ tsp.	1¼ tsp.

Cycle: Basic yeast bread. Mix the boiling water and oats and allow them to cool to room temperature, or at least to lukewarm. Then add them to the bread machine with the rest of the liquid ingredients.

Nutritional Analysis: (% Daily Value based on a 2000 calorie diet)

	Large Loaf	Small Loaf	Per serving	%D.V.
Calories:	1507	1130	79	4%
Protein (g):	43	33	2.3	-
Carbohydrate (g):	272	204	14.3	5%
Total fat (g):	26	19	1.4	2%
Saturated (g):	0	0	0	0
Cholesterol (mg):	0	0	0	0
Sodium (mg):	2030	1522	107	4%
Fiber (g):	4.8	3.6	0.3	1%

Serving size: approximately 1.1 oz.
Servings per large loaf: 19
Servings per small loaf: 15

Diabetic exchanges per serving: 1 starch/bread
Diabetic exchanges per large loaf recipe: 19 starch/bread

Wheat-free Oatmeal Bread

Ingredients:	1½ lb. loaf	1 lb. loaf
Boiling water	1 c.	¾ c.
Uncooked rolled oats or quick rolled oats	½ c.	⅜ c.
Apple juice concentrate, thawed	¼ c.	3 tbsp.
Oil	1 tbsp.	2 tsp.
Liquid lecithin (or may use additional oil)	½ tbsp.	1 tsp.
Salt	1 tsp.	¾ tsp.
White spelt flour	3 c.	2⅓ c.
Active dry yeast	2 tsp.	1½ tsp.

Cycle: Basic yeast bread. Mix the boiling water and oats and allow them to cool to room temperature, or at least to luke-warm. Then add them to the bread machine with the rest of the liquid ingredients.

Nutritional Analysis: (% Daily Value based on a 2000 calorie diet)

	Large Loaf	Small Loaf	Per serving	%D.V.
Calories:	1704	1278	81	4%
Protein (g):	58	43	2.8	-
Carbohydrate (g):	310	232	15	5%
Total fat (g):	29	22	1.4	2%
Saturated (g):	0	0	0	0
Cholesterol (mg):	0	0	0	0
Sodium (mg):	2031	1523	97	4%
Fiber (g):	10	8	0.4	1%

Serving size: approximately 1.05 oz.
Servings per large loaf: 21; Servings per small loaf: 16

Diabetic exchanges per serving: 1 starch/bread
Diabetic exchanges per large loaf recipe: 21 starch/bread

Potato Bread

Ingredients:	1½ lb. loaf	1 lb. loaf
Potato	1 small (4 oz.)	1 very small (3 oz.)
(amount in cubes)	¾ c.	½ c.
Water	¾ c.	½ c.
Additional water to bring mixture volume up to	1¼ c.	⅞ c.
Apple juice concentrate, thawed	¼ c.	3 tbsp.
Oil	1 tbsp.	2 tsp.
Liquid lecithin (or may use additional oil)	½ tbsp.	1 tsp.
Salt	1 tsp.	¾ tsp.
Bread flour	3¼ c.	2⅓ c.
Active dry yeast	1¾ tsp.	1¼ tsp.

Cycle: Basic yeast bread. Peel and cut the potato into ½" cubes. Simmer it in the first amount of water until very tender, about 25-30 minutes. Cool to lukewarm. Thoroughly mash the potatoes in the water, adding more water to bring the volume of the mixture up to the amount specified above (1¼ c. for the large loaf, ⅞ c. for the small). Add the mixture and the rest of the ingredients to the machine and start the cycle. Since potatoes vary in moisture content, you should check the consistency of this dough after 5-10 minutes of kneading and correct it if necessary. (See p. 55.)

Nutritional Analysis: (% Daily Value based on a 2000 calorie diet)

	Large Loaf	Small Loaf	Per serving	%D.V.
Calories:	1703	1192	81	4%
Protein (g):	46	32	2.2	-
Carbohydrate (g):	318	223	15	5%
Total fat (g):	24	17	1.1	2%
Saturated (g):	0	0	0	0
Cholesterol (mg):	0	0	0	0
Sodium (mg):	2036	1425	97	4%
Fiber (g):	3	2	0.1	<1%

Serving size: approximately 1.25 oz.
Servings per large loaf: 21; Servings per small loaf: 14

Diabetic exchanges per serving: 1 starch/bread
Diabetic exchanges per large loaf recipe: 21 starch/bread

Wheat-free Potato Bread

Ingredients:	1½ lb. loaf	1 lb. loaf
Potato	1 small (4 oz.)	1 very small (3 oz.)
(amount in cubes)	¾ c.	½ c.
Water	¾ c.	½ c.
Additional water to bring mixture volume up to	1¼ c.	⅞ c.
Apple juice concentrate, thawed	¼ c.	3 tbsp.
Oil	1 tbsp.	2 tsp.
Liquid lecithin (or may use additional oil)	½ tbsp.	1 tsp.
Salt	1 tsp.	¾ tsp.
White spelt flour	4 c.	2¾ c.
Active dry yeast	2¼ tsp.	1½ tsp.

Cycle: Basic yeast bread. Peel and cut the potato into ½" cubes. Simmer it in the first amount of water until very tender, about 25-30 minutes. Cool to lukewarm. Thoroughly mash the potatoes in the water, adding more water to bring the volume of the mixture up to the amount specified above (1¼ c. for the large loaf, ⅞ c. for the small). Add the mixture and the rest of the ingredients to the machine and start the cycle. Since potatoes vary in moisture content, you should check the consistency of this dough after 5-10 minutes of kneading and correct it if necessary. (See p. 55.)

Nutritional Analysis: (% Daily Value based on a 2000 calorie diet)

	Large Loaf	Small Loaf	Per serving	%D.V.
Calories:	2067	1447	80	4%
Protein (g):	69	48	2.7	-
Carbohydrate (g):	388	272	15	5%
Total fat (g):	28	20	1.1	2%
Saturated (g):	0	0	0	0
Cholesterol (mg):	0	0	0	0
Sodium (mg):	2039	1427	78	3%
Fiber (g):	10	7	0.4	2%

Serving size: approximately 1.05 oz.
Servings per large loaf: 26; Servings per small loaf: 18

Diabetic exchanges per serving: 1 starch/bread
Diabetic exchanges per large loaf recipe: 26 starch/bread

Gluten-free Rice Potato Bread

Ingredients:	1½ lb. loaf	1 lb. loaf
Water	½ c. + 1 tbsp.	½ c.
Apple juice concentrate, thawed	¼ c.	3 tbsp.
Oil	2 tbsp.	1½ tbsp.
Eggs (extra large) OR egg substitute	3 eggs or ¾ c.	2 eggs or ½ c.
Salt	1 tsp.	¾ tsp.
Vitamin C crystals	⅛ tsp.	Scant ⅛ tsp.
Guar gum	4 tsp.	3 tsp.
Brown rice flour OR white rice flour	2 c.	1½ c.
Potato flour	⅓ c.	¼ c.
Tapioca flour	⅓ c.	¼ c.
Active dry yeast	2¼ tsp.	1½ tsp.

Cycle: Basic yeast bread

Nutritional Analysis: (% Daily Value based on a 2000 calorie diet)

	Large Loaf	Small Loaf	Per serving	%D.V.
Calories (with eggs):	1891	1418	79	4%
(with egg substitute):	1883	1412	78	4%
Protein (g):	54	40	2.3	-
Carbohydrate (g):	325	244	14	5%
Total fat (g) (eggs):	52	39	2.2	3%
(with egg substitute):	61	46	2.5	4%
Saturated (g) (eggs):	5.1	3.8	0.2	<1%
(egg substitute):	0	0	0	0
Cholesterol (mg) (eggs):	1029	686	43	14%
(with egg substitute):	0	0	0	0
Sodium (mg) (eggs):	2361	1771	98	4%
(with egg substitute):	2380	1789	99	4%
Fiber (g):	17	13	0.7	2%

Serving size: approximately 1.1 oz.
Servings per large loaf: 24; Servings per small loaf: 17

Diabetic exchanges per serving: 1 starch/bread
Diabetic exchanges per large loaf recipe: 24 starch/bread

White Corn Bread

Ingredients:	1½ lb. loaf	1 lb. loaf
Water	⅞ c.	⅔ c.
Apple juice concentrate, thawed	¼ c.	3 tbsp.
Oil	1 tbsp.	2 tsp.
Liquid lecithin (or may use additional oil)	½ tbsp.	1 tsp.
Salt	1 tsp.	¾ tsp.
Bread flour	2⅞ c.	2⅛ c.
White cornmeal	⅓ c.	¼ c.
Active dry yeast	1¾ tsp.	1¼ tsp.

Cycle: Basic yeast bread

Nutritional Analysis: (% Daily Value based on a 2000 calorie diet)

	Large Loaf	Small Loaf	Per serving	%D.V.
Calories:	1590	1192	80	4%
Protein (g):	42	32	2.1	-
Carbohydrate (g):	294	221	15	5%
Total fat (g):	24	18	1.3	2%
Saturated (g):	0	0	0	0
Cholesterol (mg):	0	0	0	0
Sodium (mg):	2030	1522	107	4%
Fiber (g):	1.2	0.8	0.06	<1%

Serving size: approximately 1.15 oz.
Servings per large loaf: 20; Servings per small loaf: 15

Diabetic exchanges per serving: 1 starch/bread
Diabetic exchanges per large loaf recipe: 20 starch/bread

Wheat-free White Corn Bread

Ingredients:	1½ lb. loaf	1 lb. loaf
Water	⅞ c.	⅔ c.
Apple juice concentrate, thawed	¼ c.	3 tbsp.
Oil	1 tbsp.	2 tsp.
Liquid lecithin (or may use additional oil)	½ tbsp.	1 tsp.
Salt	1 tsp.	¾ tsp.
White spelt flour	3⅛ c. + 1 tbsp.	2⅜ c.
White cornmeal	⅓ c.	¼ c.
Active dry yeast	1¾ tsp.	1¼ tsp.

Cycle: Basic yeast bread

Nutritional Analysis: (% Daily Value based on a 2000 calorie diet)

	Large Loaf	Small Loaf	Per serving	%D.V.
Calories:	1763	1322	80	4%
Protein (g):	56	42	2.5	-
Carbohydrate (g):	299	224	14	5%
Total fat (g):	27	20	1.3	2%
Saturated (g):	0	0	0	0
Cholesterol (mg):	0	0	0	0
Sodium (mg):	2030	1522	101	4%
Fiber (g):	6.3	4.7	0.3	1%

Serving size: approximately 1.0 oz.
Servings per large loaf: 22
Servings per small loaf: 16

Diabetic exchanges per serving: 1 starch/bread
Diabetic exchanges per large loaf recipe: 22 starch/bread

Whole Grain and Extra-Nutrition Breads

Traditional Whole Wheat Bread

Ingredients:	1½ lb. loaf	1 lb. loaf
Water	1 c.	¾ c. + 1 tbsp.
Apple juice concentrate, thawed	¼ c.	3 tbsp.
Oil	1½ tbsp.	1 tbsp.
Liquid lecithin (or may use additional oil)	½ tbsp.	½ tbsp.
Salt	1 tsp.	¾ tsp.
Bread flour	1¾ c.	1⅜ c.
Whole wheat bread flour	1½ c.	1¼ c.
Active dry yeast	2 tsp.	1½ tsp.

Cycle: Basic yeast bread

Nutritional Analysis: (% Daily Value based on a 2000 calorie diet)

	Large Loaf	Small Loaf	Per serving	%D.V.
Calories:	1789	1431	81	4%
Protein (g):	60	48	2.7	-
Carbohydrate (g):	316	253	14.4	5%
Total fat (g):	34	27	1.5	2%
Saturated (g):	0	0	0	0
Cholesterol (mg):	0	0	0	0
Sodium (mg):	2034	1627	92	4%
Fiber (g):	5	4	0.25	1%

Serving size: 1.1 approximately oz.
Servings per large loaf: 22; Servings per small loaf: 18

Diabetic exchanges per serving: 1 starch/bread
Diabetic exchanges per large loaf recipe: 22 starch/bread

100% Whole Wheat Bread

Ingredients:	1½ lb. loaf	1 lb. loaf
Water	1¼ c.	1 c.
Apple juice concentrate, thawed	¼ c.	3 tbsp.
Oil	1 tbsp.	1 tbsp.
Liquid lecithin (or may use additional oil)	½ tbsp.	1 tsp.
Salt	1 tsp.	¾ tsp.
Whole wheat bread flour	3¾ c.	3 c.
Active dry yeast	2¼ tsp.	1¾ tsp.

Cycle: Basic yeast bread or whole grain

Nutritional Analysis: (% Daily Value based on a 2000 calorie diet)

	Large Loaf	Small Loaf	Per serving	%D.V.
Calories:	2111	1583	81	4%
Protein (g):	69	52	2.6	-
Carbohydrate (g):	384	288	15	5%
Total fat (g):	33	25	1.3	2%
Saturated (g):	0	0	0	0
Cholesterol (mg):	0	0	0	0
Sodium (mg):	2051	1538	79	3%
Fiber (g):	12	9	0.8	3%

Serving size: approximately 1.1 oz.
Servings per large loaf: 26
Servings per small loaf: 20

Diabetic exchanges per serving: 1 starch/bread
Diabetic exchanges per large loaf recipe: 26 starch/bread

White Wheat Bread

IF YOU OR MEMBERS OF YOUR FAMILY AR NOT REAL WHOLE WHEAT FANS, THIS MAY BE THE BREAD FOR YOU. IT IS LIGHTER IN COLOR AND FLAVOR THAN 100% WHOLE WHEAT BREAD, BUT STILL HAS ALL THE NUTRITION-AL BENEFITS OF WHOLE WHEAT.

Ingredients:	1½ lb. loaf	1 lb. loaf
Water	1¼ c.	1 c.
Apple juice concentrate, thawed	¼ c.	3 tbsp.
Oil	1 tbsp.	1 tbsp.
Liquid lecithin (or may use additional oil)	½ tbsp.	1 tsp.
Salt	1 tsp.	¾ tsp.
White whole wheat flour	3¾ c.	3 c.
Active dry yeast	2¼ tsp.	1¾ tsp.

Cycle: Basic yeast bread or whole grain

Nutritional Analysis: (% Daily Value based on a 2000 calorie diet)

	Large Loaf	Small Loaf	Per serving	%D.V.
Calories:	2111	1583	81	4%
Protein (g):	69	52	2.6	-
Carbohydrate (g):	384	288	15	5%
Total fat (g):	33	25	1.3	2%
Saturated (g):	0	0	0	0
Cholesterol (mg):	0	0	0	0
Sodium (mg):	2051	1538	79	3%
Fiber (g):	12	9	0.8	3%

Serving size: approximately 1.1 oz.
Servings per large loaf: 26
Servings per small loaf: 20

Diabetic exchanges per serving: 1 starch/bread
Diabetic exchanges per large loaf recipe: 26 starch/bread

Cracked Wheat Bread

Ingredients:	1½ lb. loaf	1 lb. loaf
Cracked wheat	¼ c.	2 tbsp.
Water	1 c.	½ c.
Water	¾ c.	½ c. + 1 tbsp.
Apple juice concentrate, thawed	3 tbsp.	2½ tbsp.
Oil	2 tsp.	1½ tsp.
Liquid lecithin (or may use additional oil)	1 tsp.	½ tsp.
Salt	¾ tsp.	½ tsp.
Cooked cracked wheat	½ c.	⅜ c.
Bread flour	2⅛ c.	1⅝ c.
Whole wheat bread flour	½ c.	⅜ c.
Active dry yeast	1¾ tsp.	1¼ tsp.

Cycle: Basic yeast bread. A few hours before or the night before making this bread, combine the uncooked cracked wheat and first amount of water listed at the top of the recipe in a saucepan, bring to a boil, reduce the heat, and simmer 15 minutes. Drain the cracked wheat thoroughly in a strainer and allow it to cool to lukewarm or room temperature. Measure the amount of cooked cracked wheat specified in the recipe and add it to the machine with the rest of the ingredients.

Nutritional Analysis: (% Daily Value based on a 2000 calorie diet)

	Large Loaf	Small Loaf	Per serving	%D.V.
Calories:	1490	1118	78	4%
Protein (g):	46	34	2.4	-
Carbohydrate (g):	281	211	15	5%
Total fat (g):	19	14	1	2%
Saturated (g):	0	0	0	0
Cholesterol (mg):	0	0	0	0
Sodium (mg):	1530	1148	81	3%
Fiber (g):	4	3	0.2	1%

Serving size: approximately 1.25 oz.;
Servings per large loaf: 19; Servings per small loaf: 14
Diabetic exchanges per serving: 1 starch/bread
Diabetic exchanges per large loaf recipe: 19 starch/bread

Cracked Spelt Bread

Ingredients:	1½ lb. programmable machine
Cracked spelt*	¼ c.
Water	1 c.

Water	¾ c.
Apple juice concentrate, thawed	¼ c.
Oil	1 tbsp.
Liquid lecithin (or use additional oil)	½ tbsp.
Salt	¾ tsp.
Cooked cracked spelt	½ c.
Whole spelt flour	½ c.
White spelt flour	2¼ c.
Active dry yeast	2 tsp.

Cycle: Welbilt ABM-150R Multi-logic cycle: Knead 2 = 20 minutes, Rise 2 = 35 minutes, Bake = 50 minutes

Cycle: Zojirushi BBCC-S15 Homemade menu cycle: Knead 1 = 10 minutes, Rest = 5 minutes, Knead 2 = 20 minutes, Rise 1 = 5 minutes, Rise 2 = 35 minutes, Bake = 50 minutes

If you cannot find cracked spelt*, process some whole spelt in a food processor or blender until it is in chunks the size of half of a spelt grain or smaller. Cook it for 30 minutes in the first amount of water listed and thoroughly drain and cool it as described in the previous recipe. Measure ½ c. of cooked cracked spelt into the machine with the rest of the ingredients.

Nutritional Analysis: (% Daily Value based on a 2000 calorie diet)

	Per Loaf	Per serving	%D.V.
Calories:	1588	79	4%
Protein (g):	54	2.7	-
Carbohydrate (g):	294	15	5%
Total fat (g):	27	1.4	2%
Saturated (g):	0	0	0
Cholesterol (mg):	0	0	0
Sodium (mg):	1531	77	3%
Fiber (g):	17	0.9	3%

Serving size: approximately 1.1 oz; Servings per loaf: 20.

Diabetic exchanges per serving: 1 starch/bread
Diabetic exchanges per whole recipe: 20 starch/bread

Whole Rye Bread

Ingredients:	1½ lb. loaf	1 lb. loaf
Water	⅓ c.	¼ c.
White grape juice	1 c.	⅔ c.
Oil	1½ tbsp.	1 tbsp.
Liquid lecithin (or may use additional oil)	½ tbsp.	½ tbsp.
Salt	1½ tsp.	1 tsp.
Unbuffered Vitamin C crystals	⅛ tsp.	Scant ⅛ tsp.
Rye flour	2½ c.	1⅔ c.
Tapioca flour	¾ c.	½ c.
Guar gum	4 tsp.	3 tsp.
Active dry yeast	2¼ tsp.	1½ tsp.

Cycle: Basic yeast bread. With some machines, you will have to assist the mixing and kneading of this dough with a spatula as described on page 58. For all machines, spread the dough evenly in the pan as soon as the last kneading time is finished.

Nutritional Analysis: (% Daily Value based on a 2000 calorie diet)

	Large Loaf	Small Loaf	Per serving	%D.V.
Calories:	1790	1193	81	4%
Protein (g):	39	26	1.7	-
Carbohydrate (g):	339	226	15	5%
Total fat (g):	31	21	1.4	2%
Saturated (g):	0	0	0	0
Cholesterol (mg):	0	0	0	0
Sodium (mg):	3023	2015	137	6%
Fiber (g):	40	27	1.8	6%

Serving size: approximately 1.1 oz.
Servings per large loaf: 22; Servings per small loaf: 15

Diabetic exchanges per serving: 1 starch/bread
Diabetic exchanges per large loaf recipe: 22 starch/bread

Light Rye Bread

Ingredients:	1½ lb. loaf	1 lb. loaf
Water	1⅛ c.	⅞ c.
Apple juice concentrate, thawed	¼ c.	3 tbsp.
Oil	1 tbsp.	2 tsp.
Liquid lecithin (or may use additional oil)	½ tbsp.	1 tsp.
Salt	1 tsp.	¾ tsp.
Caraway seed	1 tbsp.	2¼ tsp.
Bread flour	2⅝ c.	2 c.
Rye flour	1 c.	¾ c.
Active dry yeast	2 tsp.	1½ tsp.

Cycle: Basic yeast bread

Nutritional Analysis: (% Daily Value based on a 2000 calorie diet)

	Large Loaf	Small Loaf	Per serving	%D.V.
Calories:	1809	1357	82	4%
Protein (g):	51	38	2.3	-
Carbohydrate (g):	340	255	15	5%
Total fat (g):	25	19	1.1	2%
Saturated (g):	0	0	0	0
Cholesterol (mg):	0	0	0	0
Sodium (mg):	2032	1524	92	4%
Fiber (g):	17	13	0.8	3%

Serving size: approximately 1.0 oz.
Servings per large loaf: 22
Servings per small loaf: 17

Diabetic exchanges per serving: 1 starch/bread
Diabetic exchanges per large loaf recipe: 22 starch/bread

Wheat-free Light Rye Bread

Ingredients:	1½ lb. loaf	1 lb. loaf
Water	1 c.	¾ c.
Apple juice concentrate, thawed	¼ c.	3 tbsp.
Oil	1 tbsp.	2 tsp.
Liquid lecithin (or may use additional oil)	½ tbsp.	1 tsp.
Salt	1 tsp.	¾ tsp.
Caraway seed	1 tbsp.	2¼ tsp.
White spelt flour	3 c.	2¼ c.
Rye flour	1 c.	¾ c.
Active dry yeast	2 tsp.	1½ tsp.

Cycle: Basic yeast bread

Nutritional Analysis: (% Daily Value based on a 2000 calorie diet)

	Large Loaf	Small Loaf	Per serving	%D.V.
Calories:	2004	1503	83	4%
Protein (g):	65	49	2.7	-
Carbohydrate (g):	377	283	15	5%
Total fat (g):	31	23	1.3	2%
Saturated (g):	0	0	0	0
Cholesterol (mg):	0	0	0	0
Sodium (mg):	2032	1524	85	4%
Fiber (g):	22	17	0.9	3%

Serving size: approximately 1.0 oz.
Servings per large loaf: 24
Servings per small loaf: 19

Diabetic exchanges per serving: 1 starch/bread
Diabetic exchanges per large loaf recipe: 24 starch/bread

Pumpernickel Bread

Ingredients:	1½ lb. loaf	1 lb. loaf
Water	¾ c. + 1 tbsp.	⅔ c. + 1 tbsp.
Dark molasses	¼ c.	3 tbsp.
Oil	1 tbsp.	2½ tsp.
Salt	1½ tsp.	1¼ tsp.
Caraway seed	1 tbsp.	2½ tsp.
Unbuffered vitamin C crystals	⅛ tsp.	Scant ⅛ tsp.
Bread flour	1½ c.	1¼ c.
Rye flour	1¼ c.	1 c.
Carob powder	¼ c.	3 tbsp. + 1 tsp.
Active dry yeast	3 tsp.	2¼ tsp.

Cycle: Basic yeast bread. This dough is very sticky. Spread it evenly in the pan as soon as the last kneading time is finished.

Nutritional Analysis: (% Daily Value based on a 2000 calorie diet)

	Large Loaf	Small Loaf	Per serving	%D.V.
Calories:	1570	1256	79	4%
Protein (g):	62	50	3.1	-
Carbohydrate (g):	298	238	15	5%
Total fat (g):	20	16	1.0	2%
Saturated (g):	0	0	0	0
Cholesterol (mg):	0	0	0	0
Sodium (mg):	3094	2475	155	6%
Fiber (g):	21	17	1.0	3%

Serving size: approximately 1.1 oz.
Servings per large loaf: 20; Servings per small loaf: 16

Diabetic exchanges per serving: 1 starch/bread
Diabetic exchanges per large loaf recipe: 20 starch/bread

All Rye Pumpernickel Bread

Ingredients:	1½ lb. loaf	1 lb. loaf
Water	1 c.	¾ c.
Dark molasses	¼ c.	3 tbsp.
Oil	1 tbsp.	2½ tsp.
Salt	1½ tsp.	1 tsp.
Caraway seed	1 tbsp.	2½ tsp.
Unbuffered vitamin C crystals	⅛ tsp.	Scant ⅛ tsp.
White rye flour*	2¼ c.	1⅔ c. + 1 tbsp.
Rye flour	1 c.	¾ c.
Carob powder	¼ c.	3 tbsp.
Active dry yeast	3½ tsp.	2½ tsp.

Cycle: Basic yeast bread. Reserve about 1 c. of the white rye flour when you measure the ingredients into the machine and add it ¼ c. at a time during the initial kneading period. This dough is very sticky. Spread it evenly in the pan as soon as the last kneading time is finished.

*White rye flour may be purchased from the King Arthur Flour Baker's Catalogue. See "Sources," p. 236.

Nutritional Analysis: (% Daily Value based on a 2000 calorie diet)

	Large Loaf	Small Loaf	Per serving	%D.V.
Calories:	1986	1490	83	4%
Protein (g):	58	44	2.4	-
Carbohydrate (g):	438	328	18	6%
Total fat (g):	22	16	1.0	2%
Saturated (g):	0	0	0	0
Cholesterol (mg):	0	0	0	0
Sodium (mg):	3092	2319	129	5%
Fiber (g):	17	13	1.0	3%

Serving size: approximately 1.0 oz.
Servings per large loaf: 24; Servings per small loaf: 18
Diabetic exchanges per serving: 1 starch/bread
Diabetic exchanges per large loaf recipe: 24 starch/bread

Brown Bread

Ingredients:	1½ lb. or 1 lb. machine
Water	1 c.
Dark molasses	¼ c.
Oil	1 tbsp.
Liquid lecithin (or may use additional oil)	1 tsp.
Salt	1½ tsp.
Caraway seed*	1 tbsp.
White rye flour**	3½ c.
Carob powder	¼ c.
Active dry yeast	3½ tsp.

Cycle: Dough cycle. You may wish to omit the caraway seed* if you are using this recipe for a low fiber diet. This dough is very sticky, so in some machines you may need to assist the kneading with a spatula as the kneading time progresses. After the cycle finishes, remove the dough from the machine and knead it briefly on a board that has been lightly floured with white rye flour. Form it into a ball and place it on an oiled baking sheet. Slash the top of the loaf with a sharp knife and let it rise until double, 1 to 1½ hours. Bake at 375°F for 35 to 45 minutes, or until it has browned slightly and sounds hollow when tapped.

**White rye flour may be purchased from the King Arthur Flour Baker's Catalogue. See "Sources," p. 236.

Nutritional Analysis: (% Daily Value based on a 2000 calorie diet)

	Per Loaf	Per serving	%D.V.
Calories:	2026	81	4%
Protein (g):	59	2.4	-
Carbohydrate (g):	389	16	5%
Total fat (g):	26	1	2%
Saturated (g):	0	0	0
Cholesterol (mg):	0	0	0
Sodium (mg):	3093	124	5%
Fiber (g):	7	0.3	1%

Serving size: approximately 1.0 oz.; Servings per loaf: 25
Diabetic exchanges per serving: 1 starch/bread
Diabetic exchanges per whole recipe: 25 starch/bread

White Rye Bread

Ingredients:	1½ lb. loaf	1 lb. loaf
Water	⅓ c.	¼ c.
White grape juice	1 c.	¾ c.
Oil	2 tbsp.	1 tbsp.
Liquid lecithin (or may use additional oil)	1 tbsp.	2 tsp.
Salt	1 tsp.	¾ tsp.
White rye flour*	3⅞ c.	2⅞ c.
Active dry yeast	2¼ tsp.	1¾ tsp.

Cycle: Basic yeast bread. White rye dough is very sticky and may stick to the side of the pan during mixing. In some machines, you may have to use a spatula to turn the dough over and assist in the kneading, especially as the kneading time progresses. Spread the dough evenly in the pan as soon as the last kneading time is finished.

*White rye flour may be purchased from the King Arthur Flour Baker's Catalogue. See "Sources," p. 236.

Nutritional Analysis: (% Daily Value based on a 2000 calorie diet)

	Large Loaf	Small Loaf	Per serving	%D.V.
Calories:	2289	1717	82	4%
Protein (g):	60	45	2.1	-
Carbohydrate (g):	409	307	15	5%
Total fat (g):	47	35	1.7	3%
Saturated (g):	0	0	0	0
Cholesterol (mg):	0	0	0	0
Sodium (mg):	2019	1514	72	3%
Fiber (g):	7	5	0.3	1%

Serving size: approximately 0.9 oz.
Servings per large loaf: 28; Servings per small loaf: 21
Diabetic exchanges per serving: 1 starch/bread
Diabetic exchanges per large loaf recipe: 28 starch/bread

Whole Grain Spelt Bread

Ingredients:	1½ lb. loaf	1 lb. loaf
Water	1 c.	¾ c.
Apple juice concentrate, thawed	¼ c.	3 tbsp.
Oil	1 tbsp.	2 tsp.
Liquid lecithin (or may use additional oil)	½ tbsp.	1 tsp.
Salt	¾ tsp.	½ tsp.
Whole spelt flour	3⅓ c.	2½ c.
Active dry yeast	2¼ tsp.	1½ tsp.

Cycle: Basic yeast bread

Nutritional Analysis: (% Daily Value based on a 2000 calorie diet)

	Large Loaf	Small Loaf	Per serving	%D.V.
Calories:	1744	1308	79	4%
Protein (g):	56	42	2.5	-
Carbohydrate (g):	311	233	14	5%
Total fat (g):	30	23	1.4	2%
Saturated (g):	0	0	0	0
Cholesterol (mg):	0	0	0	0
Sodium (mg):	1533	1150	71	3%
Fiber (g):	27	20	1.2	5%

Serving size: approximately 1.0 oz.
Servings per large loaf: 22
Servings per small loaf: 16

Diabetic exchanges per serving: 1 starch/bread
Diabetic exchanges per large loaf recipe: 22 starch/bread

Kamut Bread

Ingredients:	1½ lb. loaf	1 lb. loaf
Water	1⅜ c.	1¼ c.
Apple juice concentrate, thawed	¼ c.	3 tbsp.
Oil	2 tbsp.	1½ tbsp.
Liquid lecithin (or may use additional oil)	1 tbsp.	½ tbsp.
Salt	1 tsp.	¾ tsp.
Kamut flour	4 c.	3¼ c.
Active dry yeast	2¾ tsp.	2¼ tsp.

Cycle: Basic yeast bread

NOTE: When making this bread in a 2 lb. machine, do not double the 1 lb. recipe. Use the 1½ lb. Recipe.

Nutritional Analysis: (% Daily Value based on a 2000 calorie diet)

	Large Loaf	Small Loaf	Per serving	%D.V.
Calories:	2445	1834	82	4%
Protein (g):	65	49	1.1	-
Carbohydrate (g):	448	336	15	5%
Total fat (g):	44	33	1.5	2%
Saturated (g):	0	0	0	0
Cholesterol (mg):	0	0	0	0
Sodium (mg):	2035	1526	68	3%
Fiber (g):	69	52	2.3	8%

Serving size: approximately 1.25 oz.
Servings per large loaf: 29
Servings per small loaf: 22

Diabetic exchanges per serving: 1 starch/bread
Diabetic exchanges per large loaf recipe: 30 starch/bread
Diabetic exchanges per small loaf recipe: 22 starch/bread

Buckwheat Bread

Ingredients:	1½ lb. programmable machine
Water	1¼ c.
Apple or pineapple juice concentrate, thawed	¼ c.
Oil	3 tbsp.
Salt	1 tsp.
Guar gum	1 tbsp.
Buckwheat flour*	2 c.
Arrowroot or tapioca flour	1¼ c.
Active dry yeast	2¼ tsp.

Cycle: Welbilt ABM-150R Multi-logic cycle: Knead 2 = 20
minutes, Rise 2 = 30 minutes, Bake = 55 minutes
Cycle: Zojirushi BBCC-S15 Homemade menu cycle:
Knead 1 = 10 minutes, Rest = 5 minutes,
Knead 2 = 20 minutes, Rise 1 = 5 minutes,
Rise 2 = 30 minutes, Bake = 55 minutes

*When using the Zojirushi, reserve 1 c. of the buckwheat flour
to add ¼ c. at a time during Knead 1 and assist the kneading
with a spatula.

Nutritional Analysis: (% Daily Value based on a 2000 calorie diet)

	Per Loaf	Per serving	%D.V.
Calories:	1754	80	4%
Protein (g):	36	1.6	-
Carbohydrate (g):	310	14	5%
Total fat (g):	42	2	3%
Saturated (g):	0	0	0
Cholesterol (mg):	0	0	0
Sodium (mg):	2029	92	4%
Fiber (g):	3	0.1	<1%

Serving size: approximately 1.2 oz.; Servings per loaf: 22
Diabetic exchanges per serving: 1 starch/bread
Diabetic exchanges per whole recipe: 22 starch/bread

Quinoa Bread

Ingredients:	1½ lb. programmable machine
Water	1 c.
Apple juice concentrate, thawed	⅓ c.
Oil	2 tbsp.
Liquid lecithin (or may use additional oil)	1 tbsp.
Salt	¾ tsp.
Cinnamon	1 tsp.
Guar gum	4 tsp.
Quinoa flour*	2½ c.
Tapioca flour	¾ c.
Active dry yeast	2¼ tsp.
Raisins (optional)	½ c.

Cycle: Welbilt ABM-150R Multi-logic cycle: Knead 2 = 20 minutes, Rise 2 = 30 minutes, Bake = 50 minutes
Cycle: Zojirushi BBCC-S15 Homemade menu cycle:
    Knead 1 = 10 minutes, Rest = 5 minutes,
    Knead 2 = 15 minutes, Rise 1 = 5 minutes,
    Rise 2 = 40-60 minutes, Bake = 50 minutes

Add the raisins 5 to 10 minutes before the end of Knead 2. *When using the Zojirushi, reserve 1 c. of the quinoa flour to add ¼ c. at a time during Knead 1 and assist the kneading with a spatula.

Nutritional Analysis: (% Daily Value based on a 2000 calorie diet)

	Per Loaf with raisins	Per Loaf without raisins	Per serving without raisins	%D.V. without raisins
Calories:	2144	1927	120	6%
Protein (g):	38	36	2.2	-
Carbohydrate (g):	443	335	21	7%
Total fat (g):	52	52	3.3	5%
Saturated (g):	0	0	0	0
Cholesterol (mg):	0	0	0	0
Sodium (mg):	1540	1538	96	4%
Fiber (g):	14	12	0.8	3%

Serving size: approximately 1.6 oz.; Servings per large loaf: 16
Diabetic exchanges per serving: 1½ starch/bread
Diabetic exchanges per whole recipe: 24 starch/bread

Amaranth Bread

Ingredients:	1½ lb. programmable machine
Water	1⅛ c.
Fruit Sweet™ or honey	3 tbsp.
Oil	2 tbsp.
Liquid lecithin (or use additional oil)	1 tbsp.
Salt	1 tsp.
Guar gum	4 tsp.
Amaranth flour*	2½ c.
Arrowroot	¾ c.
Active dry yeast	2¼ tsp.

Cycle: Welbilt ABM-150R Multi-logic cycle: Knead 2 = 20
minutes, Rise 2 = 30 minutes, Bake = 50 minutes
Cycle: Zojirushi BBCC-S15 Homemade menu cycle:
Knead 1 = 10 minutes, Rest = 5 minutes,
Knead 2 = 20 minutes, Rise 1 = 5 minutes,
Rise 2 = 30-50 minutes, Bake = 50 minutes

*When using the Zojirushi, reserve 1 c. of the amaranth flour
to add ¼ c. at a time during Knead 1 and assist the kneading
with a spatula. With either machine, spread the dough evenly
in the pan after the last kneading period.

Nutritional Analysis: (% Daily Value based on a 2000 calorie diet)

	Per Loaf	Per serving	%D.V.
Calories:	1783	81	4%
Protein (g):	39	1.8	-
Carbohydrate (g):	284	13	4%
Total fat (g):	60	27	4%
Saturated (g):	0	0	0
Cholesterol (mg):	0	0	0
Sodium (mg):	2015	92	4%
Fiber (g):	8	0.4	1%

Serving size: approximately 1.35 oz.; Servings per loaf: 22
Diabetic exchanges per serving: 1 starch/bread
Diabetic exchanges per whole recipe: 22 starch/bread

No-Egg Brown Rice Bread

Ingredients:	**1½ lb. programmable machine**
Water	1½ c.
Fruit Sweet™ or honey	3 tbsp.
Oil	2 tbsp.
Liquid lecithin (or use additional oil)	1 tbsp.
Salt	1 tsp.
Guar gum	1 tbsp.
Brown rice flour*	2¾ c.
Tapioca flour	¾ c.
Active dry yeast	2¼ tsp.

Cycle: Welbilt ABM-150R Multi-logic cycle: Knead 2 = 20
    minutes, Rise 2 = 30** minutes, Bake = 50 minutes
Cycle: Zojirushi BBCC-S15 Homemade menu cycle:
    Knead 1 = 10 minutes, Rest = 5 minutes,
    Knead 2 = 20 minutes, Rise 1 = 5 minutes,
    Rise 2 = 30** minutes, Bake = 50 minutes

*When using the Zojirushi, reserve 1 c. of the rice flour to add
¼ c. at a time during Knead 1 and assist the kneading with a
spatula. **Rise 2 should last just until the dough has barely
doubled and should end before the top of the dough begins to
collapse. With the Welbilt, the first time you make this bread
note if this point is reached before 30 minutes; if it is, use a
shorter Rise 2 the next time you make the bread.

Nutritional Analysis: (% Daily Value based on a 2000 calorie diet)

	Per Loaf	Per serving	%D.V.
Calories:	2160	83	4%
Protein (g):	36	1.4	-
Carbohydrate (g):	401	15	5%
Total fat (g):	45	2	3%
Saturated (g):	0	0	0
Cholesterol (mg):	0	0	0
Sodium (mg):	2010	77	3%
Fiber (g):	26	1.0	3%

Serving size: approximately 1.2 oz.; Servings per loaf: 26
Diabetic exchanges per serving: 1 starch/bread
Diabetic exchanges per whole recipe: 26 starch/bread

Barley Bread

Ingredients:	1½ lb. programmable machine
Water	2 c.
Fruit Sweet™ or honey	2 tbsp.
Oil	1½ tbsp.
Liquid lecithin (or use additional oil)	½ tbsp.
Salt	1 tsp.
Guar gum	3 tsp.
Barley flour*	3⅓ c.
Active dry yeast	2¼ tsp.

Cycle: Welbilt ABM-150R Multi-logic cycle: Knead 2 = 20 minutes, Rise 2 = 30 minutes, Bake = 60 minutes

Cycle: Zojirushi BBCC-S15 Homemade menu cycle: Knead 1 = 10 minutes, Rest = 5 minutes, Knead 2 = 20 minutes, Rise 1 = 5 minutes, Rise 2 = 30 minutes, Bake = 60 minutes

*When using the Zojirushi, reserve 1 c. of the barley flour to add ¼ c. at a time during Knead 1 and assist the kneading with a spatula.

Nutritional Analysis: (% Daily Value based on a 2000 calorie diet)

	Per Loaf	Per serving	%D.V.
Calories:	1787	81	4%
Protein (g):	36	1.6	-
Carbohydrate (g):	345	16	5%
Total fat (g):	30	1.4	2%
Saturated (g):	0	0	0
Cholesterol (mg):	0	0	0
Sodium (mg):	2012	91	4%
Fiber (g):	4	0.2	1%

Serving size: approximately 1.25 oz.; Servings per loaf: 22
Diabetic exchanges per serving: 1 starch/bread
Diabetic exchanges per whole recipe: 22 starch/bread

Oat Bread

Ingredients:	1½ lb. programmable machine
Water	1½ c.
Oil	2 tbsp.
Liquid lecithin (or may use additional oil)	1 tbsp.
Salt	½ tsp.
Guar gum	1 tbsp.
Date sugar	½ c.
Oat flour*	2½ c.
Arrowroot	½ c.
Active dry yeast	2¼ tsp.

Cycle: Welbilt ABM-150R Multi-logic cycle: Knead 2 = 20
        minutes, Rise 2 = 30 minutes, Bake = 50 minutes
Cycle: Zojirushi BBCC-S15 Homemade menu cycle:
        Knead 1 = 10 minutes, Rest = 5 minutes,
        Knead 2 = 20 minutes, Rise 1 = 5 minutes,
        Rise 2 = 30 minutes, Bake = 50 minutes

*When using the Zojirushi, reserve 1 c. of the oat flour to add
¼ c. at a time during Knead 1 and assist the kneading with a
spatula.

Nutritional Analysis: (% Daily Value based on a 2000 calorie diet)

	Per Loaf	Per serving	%D.V.
Calories:	1958	82	5%
Protein (g):	42	1.8	-
Carbohydrate (g):	318	13	4%
Total fat (g):	57	2.4	4%
Saturated (g):	0	0	0
Cholesterol (mg):	0	0	0
Sodium (mg):	1015	42	2%
Fiber (g):	38	1.6	5%

Serving size: approximately 1.0 oz.; Servings per loaf: 24
Diabetic exchanges per serving: 1 starch/bread
Diabetic exchanges per whole recipe: 24 starch/bread

Wheat Germ Bread

Ingredients:	1½ lb. loaf	1 lb. loaf
Water	1⅛ c.	¾ c.
Apple juice concentrate, thawed	⅜ c.	¼ c.
Oil	1½ tbsp.	2 tsp.
Liquid lecithin (or may use additional oil)	½ tbsp.	1 tsp.
Salt	1 tsp.	¾ tsp.
Bread flour	3 c.	2 c.
Whole wheat bread flour	¾ c.	½ c.
Wheat germ	⅜ c.	¼ c.
Active dry yeast	2½ tsp.	1¾ tsp.

Cycle: Basic yeast bread

Nutritional Analysis: (% Daily Value based on a 2000 calorie diet)

	Large Loaf	Small Loaf	Per serving	%D.V.
Calories:	2199	1466	81	4%
Protein (g):	65	43	2.4	-
Carbohydrate (g):	328	219	12	4%
Total fat (g):	39	26	1.4	2%
Saturated (g):	0	0	0	0
Cholesterol (mg):	0	0	0	0
Sodium (mg):	2045	1363	76	3%
Fiber (g):	4	3	0.2	1%

Serving size: approximately 1.1 oz.
Servings per large loaf: 27; Servings per small loaf: 18
Diabetic exchanges per serving: 1 starch/bread
Diabetic exchanges per large loaf recipe: 27 starch/bread

Multi-Grain Bread

Ingredients:	1½ lb. loaf	1 lb. loaf
Water	1 c.	⅔ c.
Apple juice concentrate, thawed	¼ c.	3 tbsp.
Oil	1 tbsp.	2 tsp.
Liquid lecithin (or may use additional oil)	½ tbsp.	1 tsp.
Salt	1 tsp.	¾ tsp.
Bread flour	2 c.	1⅓ c.
Whole wheat bread flour	½ c.	⅓ c.
Rye flour	¼ c.	2 tbsp. + 2 tsp.
Cornmeal	¼ c.	2 tbsp. + 2 tsp.
Cooked rice, any kind	¼ c.	2 tbsp. + 2 tsp.
Rolled oats, uncooked	¼ c.	2 tbsp. + 2 tsp.
Sunflower seeds	2 tbsp.	1 tbsp. + 1 tsp.
Sesame seeds	2 tbsp.	1 tbsp. + 1 tsp.
Active dry yeast	2¼ tsp.	1½ tsp.

Cycle: Basic yeast bread

Nutritional Analysis: (% Daily Value based on a 2000 calorie diet)

	Large Loaf	Small Loaf	Per serving	%D.V.
Calories:	1877	1251	82	4%
Protein (g):	55	37	2.4	-
Carbohydrate (g):	317	211	14	5%
Total fat (g):	44	29	2	3%
Saturated (g):	0	0	0	0
Cholesterol (mg):	0	0	0	0
Sodium (mg):	2034	1356	88	4%
Fiber (g):	12	8	0.5	2%

Serving size: approximately 1.1 oz.
Servings per large loaf: 23; Servings per small loaf: 16
Diabetic exchanges per serving: 1 starch/bread
Diabetic exchanges per large loaf recipe: 23 starch/bread

Three Seed Bread

Ingredients:	1½ lb. loaf	1 lb. loaf
Water	1 c.	¾ c.
Apple juice concentrate, thawed	¼ c.	3 tbsp.
Oil	1½ tbsp.	1 tbsp.
Liquid lecithin (or may use additional oil)	½ tbsp.	1 tsp.
Salt	1 tsp.	¾ tsp.
Bread flour	2 c.	1½ c.
Whole wheat bread flour	1 c.	¾ c.
Poppy seeds	2 tbsp.	1½ tbsp.
Sesame seeds	2 tbsp.	1½ tbsp.
Sunflower seeds	3 tbsp.	2 tbsp.
Active dry yeast	2 tsp.	1½ tsp.

Cycle: Basic yeast bread

Nutritional Analysis: (% Daily Value based on a 2000 calorie diet)

	Large Loaf	Small Loaf	Per serving	%D.V.
Calories:	1914	1435	80	4%
Protein (g):	56	42	2.3	-
Carbohydrate (g):	298	223	12	4%
Total fat (g):	57	43	2.4	4%
Saturated (g):	0	0	0	0
Cholesterol (mg):	0	0	0	0
Sodium (mg):	2037	1528	85	4%
Fiber (g):	9	7	0.4	1%

Serving size: approximately 1.0 oz.
Servings per large loaf: 24; Servings per small loaf: 18
Diabetic exchanges per serving: 1 starch/bread
Diabetic exchanges per large loaf recipe: 24 starch/bread

Pumpkin Bread

Ingredients:	1½ lb. or 1 lb. machine
Water	⅔ c.
Canned pumpkin	⅓ c.
Oil	1 tbsp.
Salt	¾ tsp.
Cinnamon	½ tsp.
Allspice	⅛ tsp.
Nutmeg	⅛ tsp.
Cloves	⅛ tsp.
Ginger	⅛ tsp.
Bread flour	2⅛ c.
Date sugar	¼ c.
Active dry yeast	1½ tsp.
- - - - - - - - - - - - - - - - - -	- - - - - - - - - - - - - - - - -
Raisins	⅓ c.

Cycle: Raisin bread cycle or basic yeast cycle. Add all of the ingredients except the raisins to the machine and start the cycle. If you are using the basic yeast cycle, set your kitchen timer to remind you to add the raisins 5 to 10 minutes before the last kneading period is finished. This dough seems to "liquify" as the cycle progresses, so you may want to scrape down the sides of the pan after the last kneading time.

Nutritional Analysis: (% Daily Value based on a 2000 calorie diet)

	Per Loaf	Per serving	%D.V.
Calories:	1306	82	4%
Protein (g):	33	2.1	-
Carbohydrate (g):	260	16	5%
Total fat (g):	16	1.1	2%
Saturated (g):	0	0	0
Cholesterol (mg):	0	0	0
Sodium (mg):	1521	95	4%
Fiber (g):	8.8	0.6	2%

Serving size: approximately 1.1 oz.; Servings per loaf: 16
Diabetic exchanges per serving: 1 starch/bread
Diabetic exchanges per whole recipe: 16 starch/bread

Wheat-free Pumpkin Bread

Ingredients:	1½ lb. programmable machine
Water	⅔ c.
Canned pumpkin	⅓ c.
Oil	1 tbsp.
Salt	¾ tsp.
Cinnamon	½ tsp.
Allspice	⅛ tsp.
Nutmeg	⅛ tsp.
Cloves	⅛ tsp.
Ginger	⅛ tsp.
White spelt flour	2⅝ c.
Date sugar	¼ c.
Active dry yeast	1¾ tsp.
Raisins	⅓ c.

Cycle: Welbilt ABM-150R Multi-logic cycle: Knead 2 = 20
    minutes, Rise 2 = 35 minutes, Bake = 50 minutes
Cycle: Zojirushi BBCC-S15 Homemade menu cycle:
    Knead 1 = 10 minutes, Rest = 5 minutes,
    Knead 2 = 20 minutes, Rise 1 = 5 minutes,
    Rise 2 = 35 minutes, Bake = 50 minutes

Add all of the ingredients except the raisins to the machine and start the cycle. Set your kitchen timer to remind you to add the raisins 5 to 10 minutes before the last kneading period is finished. This dough seems to "liquify" as the cycle progresses, so you may want to scrape down the sides of the pan after the last kneading time ends.

Nutritional Analysis: (% Daily Value based on a 2000 calorie diet)

	Per Loaf	Per serving	%D.V.
Calories:	1548	81	4%
Protein (g):	47	2.5	-
Carbohydrate (g):	305	16	5%
Total fat (g):	19	1.0	2%
Saturated (g):	0	0	0
Cholesterol (mg):	0	0	0
Sodium (mg):	1521	80	3%
Fiber (g):	13	0.7	2%

Serving size: approximately 1.0 oz.; Servings per loaf: 19
Diabetic exchanges per serving: 1 starch/bread
Diabetic exchanges per whole recipe: 19 starch/bread

Protein Bread

THIS BREAD IS UNUSUAL, BUT TASTY, AND MAY BE USEFUL TO THOSE ON LOW CARBOHYDRATE OR HYPOGLYCEMIC DIETS.

Ingredients:	1½ lb. loaf	1 lb. loaf
Water	1 c.	⅔ c.
Apple juice concentrate, thawed	¼ c.	2 tbsp. + 2 tsp.
Oil	1 tbsp.	2 tsp.
Salt	1 tsp.	¾ tsp.
Gluten flour	1 c.	⅔ c.
Soy flour	1 c.	⅔ c.
Wheat germ	¾ c.	½ c.
Active dry yeast	1½ tsp.	1 tsp.

Cycle: Basic yeast bread

Nutritional Analysis: (% Daily Value based on a 2000 calorie diet)

	Large Loaf	Small Loaf	Per serving	%D.V.
Calories:	1449	966	80	4%
Protein (g):	149	99	8.3	-
Carbohydrate (g):	126	84	7	2%
Total fat (g):	39	26	2.2	3%
Saturated (g):	0	0	0	0
Cholesterol (mg):	0	0	0	0
Sodium (mg):	2108	1405	117	5%
Fiber (g):	4	3	0.3	1%

Serving size: approximately 1.0 oz.
Servings per large loaf: 18; Servings per small loaf: 12

Diabetic exchanges per serving: ½ starch/bread + ½ lean meat
Diabetic exchanges per large loaf recipe: 9 starch/bread + 9 lean meat

Corny Bread

Ingredients:	1½ lb. loaf	1 lb. loaf
Water	⅞ c.	⅔ c.
Apple juice concentrate, thawed	¼ c.	3 tbsp.
Oil	1 tbsp.	2 tsp.
Liquid lecithin (or may use additional oil)	½ tbsp.	1 tsp.
Salt	1 tsp.	¾ tsp.
Bread flour	2¾ c.	2 c. + 1 tbsp.
Cornmeal (yellow)	⅓ c.	¼ c.
Active dry yeast	1¾ tsp.	1¼ tsp.

Cycle: Basic yeast bread

Nutritional Analysis: (% Daily Value based on a 2000 calorie diet)

	Large Loaf	Small Loaf	Per serving	%D.V.
Calories:	1540	1155	81	4%
Protein (g):	41	31	2.2	-
Carbohydrate (g):	283	212	15	5%
Total fat (g):	24	18	1.3	2%
Saturated (g):	0	0	0	0
Cholesterol (mg):	0	0	0	0
Sodium (mg):	2030	1522	107	4%
Fiber (g):	1.1	0.8	0.06	<1%

Serving size: approximately 1.15 oz.
Servings per large loaf: 19; Servings per small loaf: 14

Diabetic exchanges per serving: 1 starch/bread
Diabetic exchanges per large loaf recipe: 19 starch/bread

Wheat-free Corny Bread

Ingredients:	1½ lb. loaf	1 lb. loaf
Water	⅞ c.	⅔ c.
Apple juice concentrate, thawed	¼ c.	3 tbsp.
Oil	1 tbsp.	2 tsp.
Liquid lecithin (or may use additional oil)	½ tbsp.	1 tsp.
Salt	1 tsp.	¾ tsp.
White spelt flour	3 c.	2¼ c.
Cornmeal (yellow)	⅓ c.	¼ c.
Active dry yeast	1¾ tsp.	1¼ tsp.

Cycle: Basic yeast bread

Nutritional Analysis: (% Daily Value based on a 2000 calorie diet)

	Large Loaf	Small Loaf	Per serving	%D.V.
Calories:	1685	1264	84	4%
Protein (g):	53	40	2.7	-
Carbohydrate (g):	283	212	14	5%
Total fat (g):	27	20	1.3	2%
Saturated (g):	0	0	0	0
Cholesterol (mg):	0	0	0	0
Sodium (mg):	2030	1522	101	4%
Fiber (g):	6	5	0.3	1%

Serving size: approximately 1.1 oz.
Servings per large loaf: 20; Servings per small loaf: 15

Diabetic exchanges per serving: 1 starch/bread
Diabetic exchanges per large loaf recipe: 20 starch/bread

Gluten-free Corny Bread

Ingredients:	1½ lb. loaf	1 lb. loaf
Water	½ c.	⅓ c.
Apple juice concentrate, thawed	¼ c.	3 tbsp.
Oil	2 tbsp.	1 tbsp. + 1 tsp.
Eggs (extra large) OR egg substitute	3 eggs or ¾ c.	2 eggs or ½ c.
Salt	1 tsp.	¾ tsp.
Vitamin C crystals	⅛ tsp.	Scant ⅛ tsp.
Guar gum	4 tsp.	3 tsp.
Brown rice flour	1⅔ c.	1⅛ c.
Cornmeal (yellow)	⅓ c.	¼ c.
Potato flour	⅓ c.	¼ c.
Tapioca flour	⅓ c.	¼ c.
Active dry yeast	2¼ tsp.	1½ tsp.

Cycle: Basic yeast bread

Nutritional Analysis: (% Daily Value based on a 2000 calorie diet)

	Large Loaf	Small Loaf	Per serving	%D.V.
Calories (with eggs):	1486	1114	82	4%
(with egg substitute):	1478	1108	82	4%
Protein (g):	53	40	2.9	-
Carbohydrate (g):	318	238	17	6%
Total fat (g) (eggs):	53	40	2.9	4%
(with egg substitute):	62	46	3.2	5%
Saturated (g) (eggs):	5.1	3.8	0.3	1%
(egg substitute):	0	0	0	0
Cholesterol (mg) (eggs):	1029	686	57	19%
(with egg substitute):	0	0	0	0
Sodium (mg) (eggs):	2361	1771	98	4%
(with egg substitute):	2286	1714	127	5%
Fiber (g):	14	11	0.8	3%

Serving size: approximately 1.3 oz.
Servings per large loaf: 18; Servings per small loaf: 14
Diabetic exchanges per serving: 1 starch/bread
Diabetic exchanges per large loaf recipe: 18 starch/bread

Bread of Gold

Ingredients:	1½ lb. loaf	1 lb. loaf
Water	1 c.	⅔ c.
Apple juice concentrate, thawed	¼ c.	2½ tbsp.
Oil	1½ tbsp.	1 tbsp.
Liquid lecithin (or may use additional oil)	½ tbsp.	1 tsp.
Salt	1 tsp.	¾ tsp.
Bread flour	1¾ c.	1⅛ c. + 1 tbsp.
Kamut flour	1½ c.	1 c.
Active dry yeast	2¼ tsp.	1½ tsp.

Cycle: Basic yeast bread

Nutritional Analysis: (% Daily Value based on a 2000 calorie diet)

	Large Loaf	Small Loaf	Per serving	%D.V.
Calories:	1731	1154	79	4%
Protein (g):	47	31	2.1	-
Carbohydrate (g):	315	209	14.3	5%
Total fat (g):	31	21	1.4	2%
Saturated (g):	0	0	0	0
Cholesterol (mg):	0	0	0	0
Sodium (mg):	2030	1353	92	4%
Fiber (g):	24	16	1.1	4%

Serving size: 1.1 approximately oz.
Servings per large loaf: 22
Servings per small loaf: 15

Diabetic exchanges per serving: 1 starch/bread
Diabetic exchanges per large loaf: 22 starch/bread

Wheat-free Bread of Gold

Ingredients:	1½ lb. loaf	1 lb. loaf
Water	1 c.	⅔ c.
Apple juice concentrate, thawed	¼ c.	2½ tbsp.
Oil	1½ tbsp.	1 tbsp.
Liquid lecithin (or may use additional oil)	½ tbsp.	1 tsp.
Salt	1 tsp.	¾ tsp.
White spelt flour	2⅛ c.	1⅜ c.
Kamut flour	1½ c.	1 c.
Active dry yeast	2¼ tsp.	1½ tsp.

Cycle: Basic yeast bread

Nutritional Analysis: (% Daily Value based on a 2000 calorie diet)

	Large Loaf	Small Loaf	Per serving	%D.V.
Calories:	1913	1275	80	4%
Protein (g):	58	39	2.4	-
Carbohydrate (g):	351	234	15	5%
Total fat (g):	33	22	1.4	2%
Saturated (g):	0	0	0	0
Cholesterol (mg):	0	0	0	0
Sodium (mg):	2030	1353	85	4%
Fiber (g):	28	19	1.2	4%

Serving size: approximately 1.0 oz.
Servings per large loaf: 24
Servings per small loaf: 16

Diabetic exchanges per serving: 1 starch/bread
Diabetic exchanges per large loaf: 24 starch/bread

Sourdough and Variety Breads

ALL ABOUT SOURDOUGH

What is sourdough? It is yeast bread that is leavened by a sourdough starter, or culture, rather than by commercial baker's yeast. The culture contains wild yeast, which produces gas and causes the bread to rise, and bacteria of the genus *Lactobacillus* that give the bread a sour flavor. There are many different sourdough cultures, each with a special flavor of its own and unique rising characteristics.

Perhaps the use of sourdough cultures is beyond the scope of a book dedicated to making bread as easily as possible. However, there are some people who are allergic to commercial baker's yeast and bread made with it who seem to tolerate sourdough bread. Sourdough bread is <u>not</u> yeast-free; maybe these people are not allergic to the wild yeast but are to baker's yeast, much as one may be allergic to lettuce but not to endive. If you are allergic to yeast, be sure to ask your doctor before trying sourdough bread.

Another reason to consider making sourdough bread is the flavor of the bread itself. If you have eaten at Fisherman's Wharf in San Francisco and are a fan of the sourdough bread there, you may consider the time spent maintaining and using a sourdough culture worthwhile when you taste how delicious your bread can be.

Some cookbooks contain recipes for making your own sourdough starter. However, in the process of catching and growing wild yeasts from your environment, you may also catch some molds and bacteria that you would rather not have. The flavor of bread made from homemade starters is barely sour. If you want to make sourdough bread that tastes like "the real thing" from Fisherman's Wharf, purchase a San Francisco sourdough starter from Sourdoughs International, Inc. (see "Sources," p. 238). For the best flavor, use it alone in your sourdough bread; never use commercial baker's yeast with it.

Your culture from Sourdoughs International will come with detailed instructions on how to activate and maintain it. Activating it involves "feeding" it with flour and water several times and keeping it warm. The dried sourdough culture you receive contains a small amount (less than ¼ c.) of wheat flour. If you wish to make wheat-free bread, feed your culture with white spelt flour. When I activated my cultures, I fed them with white spelt flour nine times before using them in bread. Sparing you the arithmetic, this meant that there was about ⅟₃₂ tsp. of wheat flour per cup of starter by the time it was first used, or about ⅟₁₆ tsp. in a large loaf of bread weighing about 2 lbs. With repeated use and feeding of the culture, the amount of wheat flour continues to decrease, so now, over a year later, I consider my starters to be essentially wheat-free. However, if you are very sensitive to wheat, the flour in the purchased culture may be a problem.

Sourdough bread is a challenge to the bread machine baker because wild yeast takes much longer to leaven bread than commercial baker's yeast and bread machine cycles are based on the way baker's yeast leavens bread. Sourdough is also not well adapted to bread machine cycles because the *lactobacilli* take about 12 hours to develop the full flavor you want in your bread. Also, sourdough cultures are unpredictable, behaving differently from one use to the next. I find it best to use the dough cycle of my bread machine to make the dough and allow the bread to rise outside of the machine where I can easily judge when it is ready to be baked. For further information about sourdough and sourdough bread machine baking, refer to *Worldwide Sourdoughs From Your Bread Machine* by Donna German and Ed Wood.

Classic San Francisco Sourdough Bread

Ingredients:	1½ lb. machine	1 lb. machine
Sourdough culture	2 c.	1⅓ c.
Bread flour	1½ c.	1 c.
Salt	1 tsp.	¾ tsp
Bread flour	2 to 2¾ c.	1⅓ to 1⅞ c.

Cycle: Dough cycle. The night before you want to make bread, mix the culture and the first amount of flour in a glass, plastic, or ceramic mixing bowl. (Do not use a metal bowl.) If your bread machine pan does not have a hole in the bottom, you may mix them in your bread machine pan in the machine. Then cover the bowl or bread machine pan with plastic wrap or a towel and put it in a warm place overnight. (If you made a "proofing box" to activate your culture, this is an ideal place.) In the morning, put the pan back into the machine or transfer the mixture in the bowl to your machine pan. Add the salt and the smallest amount of the second flour listing above, and start the dough cycle. After mixing, remove the dough from the pan and knead in enough of the remaining flour so the dough is no longer sticky. Shape it into either a round or long loaf and put it on a baking sheet that has been liberally sprinkled with cornmeal. Slash the top of the loaf and put it in a warm place to rise until doubled, about 3 to 5 hours. Preheat your oven to 375°F. Spray the loaf with water before baking and at 5 and 10 minutes into the baking time. If desired, bake a few potatoes along with the bread for added moisture to make the crust crisp. Bake for 65 to 80 minutes, or until brown.

Nutritional Analysis: (% Daily Value based on a 2000 calorie diet)

	Large Loaf	Small Loaf	Per serving	%D.V.
Calories:	1733	1155	79	4%
Protein (g):	56	37	2.5	-
Carbohydrate (g):	355	237	16	5%
Total fat (g):	5	3	0.2	<1%
Saturated (g):	0	0	0	0
Cholesterol (mg):	0	0	0	0
Sodium (mg):	2010	1340	72	3%
Fiber (g):	2	1	0.1	<1%

Serving size: approximately 1.3 oz.
Servings per large loaf: 22; Serving per small loaf: 15
Diabetic exchanges per serving: 1 starch/bread

Wheat-free San Francisco Sourdough Bread

Ingredients:	1½ lb. machine	1 lb. machine
White spelt sourdough culture (see p. 111)	2 c.	1⅓ c.
White spelt flour	1½ c.	1 c.
Salt	1 tsp.	¾ tsp
White spelt flour	2½ to 3¾ c.	1⅔ to 2½ c.

Cycle: Dough cycle. The night before you want to make bread, mix the culture and the first amount of flour in a glass, plastic, or ceramic mixing bowl. (Do not use a metal bowl.) If your bread machine pan does not have a hole in the bottom, you may mix them in your bread machine pan in the machine. Then cover the bowl or bread machine pan with plastic wrap or a towel and put it in a warm place overnight. (If you made a "proofing box" to activate your culture, this is an ideal place.) In the morning, put the pan back into the machine or transfer the mixture in the bowl to your machine pan. Add the salt and the smallest amount of the second flour listing above, and start the dough cycle. After mixing, remove the dough from the pan and knead in enough of the remaining flour so the dough is no longer sticky. Shape it into either a round or long loaf and put it on a baking sheet that has been liberally sprinkled with cornmeal or white spelt flour. Slash the top of the loaf and put it in a warm place to rise until doubled, about 3 to 5 hours. Preheat your oven to 375°F. Spray the loaf with water before baking and at 5 and 10 minutes into the baking time. If desired, bake a few potatoes along with the bread for added moisture to make the crust crisp. Bake for 65 to 80 minutes, or until brown.

Nutritional Analysis: (% Daily Value based on a 2000 calorie diet)

	Large Loaf	Small Loaf	Per serving	%D.V.
Calories:	2144	1429	77	4%
Protein (g):	83	55	3.0	-
Carbohydrate (g):	434	289	16	5%
Total fat (g):	10	7	0.4	<1%
Saturated (g):	0	0	0	0
Cholesterol (mg):	0	0	0	0
Sodium (mg):	2010	1340	72	3%
Fiber (g):	10	7	0.4	1%

Serving size: approximately 1.2 oz.
Servings per large loaf: 28; Servings per small loaf: 18
Diabetic exchanges per serving: 1 starch/bread

Easy Sour Rye Bread

Ingredients:	1½ lb. loaf	1 lb. loaf
Water	1 c.	¾ c.
Apple juice concentrate, thawed	¼ c.	3 tbsp.
Oil	1 tbsp.	2 tsp.
Liquid lecithin (or may use additional oil)	½ tbsp.	1 tsp.
Salt	1½ tsp.	1 tsp.
Caraway seed (optional)	1 tbsp.	2¼ tsp.
Heidelberg rye sour*	2 tbsp.	1½ tbsp.
Bread flour	2¼ c.	1⅔ c.
Rye flour	1 c.	¾ c.
Active dry yeast	2¼ tsp.	1¾ tsp.

Cycle: Basic yeast bread

*Heidelberg rye sour may be purchased from the King Arthur Flour Baker's Catalogue. See "Sources," p. 235.

Nutritional Analysis: (% Daily Value based on a 2000 calorie diet)

	Large Loaf	Small Loaf	Per serving	%D.V.
Calories:	1706	1280	81	4%
Protein (g):	25	19	1.1	-
Carbohydrate (g):	319	239	15	5%
Total fat (g):	24	18	1.1	2%
Saturated (g):	0	0	0	0
Cholesterol (mg):	0	0	0	0
Sodium (mg):	3032	2274	144	6%
Fiber (g):	17	13	1	3%

Serving size: approximately 1.15 oz.
Servings per large loaf: 21; Servings per small loaf: 16
Diabetic exchanges per serving: 1 starch/bread

Wheat-free Easy Sour Rye Bread

Ingredients:	1½ lb. loaf	1 lb. loaf
Water	1 c.	¾ c.
Apple juice concentrate, thawed	¼ c.	3 tbsp.
Oil	1 tbsp.	2 tsp.
Liquid lecithin (or may use additional oil)	½ tbsp.	1 tsp.
Salt	1½ tsp.	1 tsp.
Caraway seed (optional)	1 tbsp.	2¼ tsp.
Heidelberg rye sour*	2 tbsp.	1½ tbsp.
White spelt flour	2¾ c.	2 c. + 1 tbsp.
Rye flour	1 c.	¾ c.
Active dry yeast	2¼ tsp.	1¾ tsp.

Cycle: Basic yeast bread

*Heidelberg rye sour may be purchased from the King Arthur Flour Baker's Catalogue. See "Sources," p. 235.

Nutritional Analysis: (% Daily Value based on a 2000 calorie diet)

	Large Loaf	Small Loaf	Per serving	%D.V.
Calories:	1947	1460	81	4%
Protein (g):	63	47	2.6	-
Carbohydrate (g):	365	274	15	5%
Total fat (g):	28	21	1.2	2%
Saturated (g):	0	0	0	0
Cholesterol (mg):	0	0	0	0
Sodium (mg):	3033	2275	126	5%
Fiber (g):	22	17	1	3%

Serving size: approximately 1.1 oz.
Servings per large loaf: 24; Servings per small loaf: 18
Diabetic exchanges per serving: 1 starch/bread

Seeded Bread
Braid or Ring

Ingredients: 1½ lb. or 1 lb. machine

One 1½ lb. loaf batch of dough for any basic bread, pages 61
      to 75 or 77 to 78, or any whole-grain bread, pages
      79 to 92, 99 to 101, 105 to 106 or 108 to 109.
Bread wash, p. 129, OR 1 egg white, slightly beaten
Your choice of two of the following:
      1½ tbsp. sesame seeds
      1½ tbsp. poppy seeds
      2 tbsp. wheat germ

Cycle: Dough cycle. Put the ingredients for the type of bread
you have chosen into your machine and run the dough cycle.
When it is finished, for a braid, divide the dough into three
parts and roll each into a 15″ rope. Lay them on an oiled baking sheet and braid them. For a ring, divide the dough into two
parts and roll each part into a 20″ to 24″ rope. Place the ropes
side by side near one edge of an oiled baking sheet. Bring the
outer rope across the inner one repeatedly until the ropes are
formed into a ring-shaped twist. Pinch the ends of the ring
together. Let the loaf rise until double, about 40 to 60 minutes.
Brush it with the wash or egg. Sprinkle one type of seed or the
wheat germ on one section of the twist or braid and another on
the next, alternating types. Bake at 375°F for 35 to 45 minutes,
covering the loaf with foil for the last 10 minutes if needed to
prevent over-browning.

Nutritional Analysis: To the whole loaf values for the recipe used add 105 calories,
7 grams of protein, 12 grams of carbohydrate, 7 grams of fat, and 1 mg. of sodium.

Serving size and servings per loaf: Same as for the bread recipe used
Diabetic exchanges per serving: Same as for the bread recipe used

Onion Dill Bread

Ingredients:	1½ lb. loaf	1 lb. loaf
One batch of any white bread, pages 61 to 78, or any whole grain bread, pages 79 to 84 or 90 to 99	1½ lb. amounts of all ingredients	1 lb. amounts of all ingredients
Dry minced onion	2 tsp.	1½ tsp.
Dry dill	2 tsp.	1½ tsp.

Cycle: Basic yeast bread cycle or dough cycle, same as in the recipe you are using. When you add the bread ingredients to the bread machine pan, add the onion and dill with the salt.

Nutritional analysis: Same as for the recipe used
Serving size and servings per loaf: Same as for the bread recipe used
Diabetic exchanges per serving: Same as for the bread recipe used

Italian Herb Bread

Ingredients:	1½ lb. loaf	1-lb loaf
One batch of any white bread, pages 61 to 78, or any whole grain bread, pages 79 to 84 or 90 to 99	1½ lb. amounts of all ingredients	1 lb. amounts of all ingredents
Sweet basil, dry OR fresh	2 tsp. dry OR 2 tbsp. fresh	1½ tsp. dry OR 1½ tbsp. fresh
Oregano, dry OR fresh	2 tsp. dry OR 2 tbsp. fresh	1½ tsp. dry OR 1½ tbsp. fresh

Cycle: Basic yeast bread cycle or dough cycle, same as in the recipe you are using. When you add the bread ingredients to the bread machine pan, add the herbs with the salt.

Nutritional analysis: Same as for the recipe used
Serving size and servings per loaf: Same as for the bread recipe used

Diabetic exchanges per serving: Same as for the bread recipe used

Poppy Seed Bread

Ingredients:	1½ lb. loaf	1 lb. loaf
One batch of any white bread, pages 61 to 78, or any whole grain bread, pages 79 to 84 or 90 to 99	1½ lb. amounts of all ingredients	1 lb. amounts of all ingredients
Poppy seeds	2 tbsp.	1½ tbsp.

Cycle: Basic yeast bread cycle or dough cycle, same as in the recipe you are using. When you add the bread ingredients to the bread machine pan, add the poppy seeds with the salt

Nutritional analysis: To the whole-loaf values for the recipe used, add:

> 1½ lb. loaf: 80 calories, 4 g. protein, 7 g. carbohydrate,
> 13 g. fat, 3 mg. sodium, and 5 g. fiber
> 1 lb. loaf: 60 calories, 3 g. protein, 5 g. carbohydrate,
> 9 g. fat, 2 mg. sodium, and 3 g. fiber

The per serving values and % Daily Value are essentially the same as for the recipe used.
Serving size and servings per loaf: Same as for the bread recipe used
Diabetic exchanges per serving: Same as for the bread recipe used

Blueberry Bread

Ingredients:	1½ lb. loaf	1 lb. loaf
One batch of any white bread, pages 61 to 78, or any whole grain bread, pages 79 to 84 or 90 to 99	1½ lb. amounts of all ingredients	1 lb. amounts of all ingredients
Dry blueberries	½ c.	⅓ c.

Cycle: Basic yeast bread or raisin bread cycle. Add the blueberries at the "beep" in the raisin bread cycle or 5 to 10 minutes before the last kneading ends in the basic yeast bread cycle.

Nutritional analysis: To the whole-loaf values for the recipe used, add:
> 1½ lb. loaf: 218 calories, 2.5 g. protein, 52 g. carbohydrate, 2 g. fat,
> 5 mg. sodium, and 5 g. fiber
> 1 lb. loaf: 145 calories, 1.5 g. protein, 35 g. carbohydrate, 1 g. fat,
> 3 mg. sodium, and 3 g. fiber

To the calories per serving, add 8-10 calories. To the carbohydrate per serving add 2 g. The rest of the per serving values and the % Daily Value are essentially the same as for the recipe used.

Serving size and servings per loaf: Same as for the bread recipe used
Diabetic exchanges per serving: Same as for the bread recipe used

Chili Corn Bread

Ingredients:	1½ lb. loaf	1 lb. loaf
Water	⅝ c.	⅜ c.
Apple juice concentrate, thawed	¼ c.	3 tbsp.
4 oz. cans mild green chilies	1	1
Oil	1 tbsp.	2 tsp.
Liquid lecithin (or may use additional oil)	½ tbsp.	1 tsp.
Salt	1 tsp.	¾ tsp.
Bread flour	2⅞ c.	2⅛ c. + 1 tbsp.
Cornmeal	⅓ c.	¼ c.
Active dry yeast	1¾ tsp.	1¼ tsp.

Cycle: Basic yeast bread

Nutritional Analysis: (% Daily Value based on a 2000 calorie diet)

	Large Loaf	Small Loaf	Per serving	%D.V.
Calories:	1630	1223	81	4%
Protein (g):	42	32	2.1	-
Carbohydrate (g):	304	228	15	5%
Total fat (g):	24	18	1.2	2%
Saturated (g):	0	0	0	0
Cholesterol (mg):	0	0	0	0
Sodium (mg):	2190	1643	110	5%
Fiber (g):	1.3	1	0.07	<1%

Serving size: approximately 1.2 oz.
Servings per large loaf: 20
Servings per small loaf: 15

Diabetic exchanges per serving: 1 starch/bread

Wheat-free Chili Corn Bread

Ingredients:	1½ lb. loaf	1 lb. loaf
Water	⅝ c.	⅜ c.
Apple juice concentrate, thawed	¼ c.	3 tbsp.
4 oz. cans mild green chilies	1	1
Oil	1 tbsp.	2 tsp.
Liquid lecithin (or may use additional oil)	½ tbsp.	1 tsp.
Salt	1 tsp.	¾ tsp.
White spelt flour	3⅛ c.	2⅓ c.
Cornmeal	⅓ c.	¼ c.
Active dry yeast	1¾ tsp.	1¼ tsp.

Cycle: Basic yeast bread

Nutritional Analysis: (% Daily Value based on a 2000 calorie diet)

	Large Loaf	Small Loaf	Per serving	%D.V.
Calories:	1777	1333	81	4%
Protein (g):	55	41	2.5	-
Carbohydrate (g):	331	248	15	5%
Total fat (g):	27	20	1.2	2%
Saturated (g):	0	0	0	0
Cholesterol (mg):	0	0	0	0
Sodium (mg):	2190	1643	100	4%
Fiber (g):	6.3	4.7	0.3	1%

Serving size: approximately 1.15 oz.
Servings per large loaf: 22
Servings per small loaf: 17

Diabetic exchanges per serving: 1 starch/bread

Herb Focaccia

Ingredients:

One batch of "Italian Bread" dough
  OR "Wheat-free Italian Bread" dough, pages 65 to 66
4 tsp. olive oil
2-3 tbsp. minced fresh sweet basil or rosemary
  OR 2-3 tsp. dry sweet basil or rosemary

Cycle: Dough cycle, using only the Italian bread ingredients, not the oil and herbs. When the cycle is finished, remove the dough from the machine and divide it in half. Spray two baking sheets with a cooking oil spray or oil them lightly. Roll out each piece of dough on a baking sheet to an 8″ to 10″ circle, about ½″ thick. Brush each circle with 2 tsp. of olive oil and sprinkle with the herbs. Let rise in a warm place for 30 minutes or until double in volume. Bake at 375°F for 20 to 25 minutes, or until brown. Cut into wedges to serve.

Nutritional Analysis: To the values for a whole loaf of Italian bread add 160 calories and 18 grams of fat.

Serving size: Same as for the bread recipe used

Diabetic exchanges per whole batch: Same number of starch/bread exchanges as for the whole bread recipe used + 4 fat exchanges

Salt and Pepper Focaccia

Make as for "Herb Focaccia," above, except substitute ½ tsp. kosher salt and ¼ tsp. pepper for the herbs.

Nutritional Analysis: To the values for a whole loaf of Italian bread add 160 calories, 18 grams of fat, and 1000 mg. of sodium.

Serving size: Same as for the bread recipe used

Diabetic exchanges per whole batch: Same number of starch/bread exchanges as for the whole bread recipe used + 4 fat exchanges

Pita Bread

Ingredients:

One batch of bread dough
for White Bread, page 61, 1 ½ lb. loaf

Cycle: Dough cycle. After the cycle is finished, remove the
dough from the machine and preheat your oven to 475°F. Roll
the dough out on a very lightly oiled board with an oiled rolling
pin to about ¼″ thickness. Fold the dough in half and roll it to
¼″ thickness again. Fold and roll it repeatedly until you have
rolled it 15 to 20 times, letting the dough "rest" for five minutes after each five rollings. Divide the dough into eight pieces,
and allow the dough to rest for five minutes. Roll each piece out
into a 6″ to 7″ circle, flouring both sides of the circle as you roll
it. Place the pita breads on lightly floured baking sheets and
bake them in the preheated oven until they are lightly browned,
about 3 to 9 minutes. Remove them from the oven and immediately wrap them in a very lightly dampened dishcloth. When
they are completely cool, remove them from the dishcloth and
store them in a plastic bag. Use a serrated knife to cut them in
half and open any places where the top and bottom of the pita
did not separate.

Nutritional Analysis: (% Daily Value based on a 2000 calorie diet)

	Per batch	Per pita	%D.V.
Calories:	1557	195	10%
Protein (g):	43	5.4	-
Carbohydrate (g):	286	36	12%
Total fat (g):	23	2.8	4%
Saturated (g):	0	0	0
Cholesterol (mg):	0	0	0
Sodium (mg):	2031	254	11%
Fiber (g):	0.9	0.1	<1%

Serving size: one pita bread
Servings per batch: eight pita breads

Diabetic exchanges per serving: 2½ starch/bread

White Spelt Pita Bread

Ingredients:

One batch of bread dough for
  White Spelt Bread, page 63, 1½ lb. loaf

Cycle: Dough cycle. After the cycle is finished, remove the dough from the machine and preheat your oven to 475°F. Roll the dough out on a very lightly oiled board with an oiled rolling pin to about ¼" thickness. Fold the dough in half and roll it to ¼" thickness again. Fold and roll it repeatedly until you have rolled it 15 to 20 times. Divide the dough into eight pieces. Roll each piece out into a 6" to 7" circle, flouring both sides of the circle as you roll it. Place the pita breads on lightly floured baking sheets and bake them in the preheated oven until they are lightly browned, about 3 to 7 minutes. Remove them from the oven and immediately wrap them in a very lightly dampened dishcloth. When they are completely cool, remove them from the dishcloth and store them in a plastic bag. Use a serrated knife to cut them in half and open any places where the top and bottom of the pita did not separate.

Nutritional Analysis: (% Daily Value based on a 2000 calorie diet)

	Per batch	Per pita	%D.V.
Calories:	1432	179	9%
Protein (g):	48	6	-
Carbohydrate (g):	265	33	11%
Total fat (g):	21	2.6	4%
Saturated (g):	0	0	0
Cholesterol (mg):	0	0	0
Sodium (mg):	1526	191	8%
Fiber (g):	6	0.7	2%

Serving size: one pita bread
Servings per batch: 8 pita breads

Diabetic exchanges per serving: 2¼ starch/bread

Whole Wheat Pita Bread

Ingredients:

One batch of bread dough for
    100% Whole Wheat Bread, page 80, 1½ lb. loaf

Cycle: Dough cycle. After the cycle is finished, remove the dough from the machine and preheat your oven to 475°F. Roll the dough out on a very lightly oiled board with an oiled rolling pin to about ¼″ thickness. Fold the dough in half and roll it to ¼″ thickness again. Fold and roll it repeatedly until you have rolled it 15 to 20 times. Divide the dough into ten pieces. Roll each piece out into a 5″ to 6″ circle, flouring both sides of the circle as you roll it. Place the pita breads on lightly floured baking sheets and bake them in the preheated oven until they are lightly browned, about 7 to 11 minutes. Remove them from the oven and immediately wrap them in a very lightly dampened dishcloth. When they are completely cool, remove them from the dishcloth and store them in a plastic bag. Use a serrated knife to cut them in half and open any places where the top and bottom of the pita did not separate.

Nutritional Analysis: (% Daily Value based on a 2000 calorie diet)

	Per batch	Per pita	%D.V.
Calories:	2111	211	11%
Protein (g):	69	7	-
Carbohydrate (g):	384	38	13%
Total fat (g):	33	3.3	5%
Saturated (g):	0	0	0
Cholesterol (mg):	0	0	0
Sodium (mg):	2051	205	9%
Fiber (g):	12	1.2	4%

Serving size: one pita bread
Servings per batch: 10 pita breads

Diabetic exchanges per serving: 2½ starch/bread

Whole Spelt Pita Bread

Ingredients:

One batch of bread dough for
  Whole Grain Spelt Bread, page 91, 1½ lb. loaf

Cycle: Dough cycle. After the cycle is finished, remove the dough from the machine and preheat your oven to 475°F. Roll the dough out on a very lightly oiled board with an oiled rolling pin to about ¼" thickness. Fold the dough in half and roll it to ¼" thickness again. Fold and roll it repeatedly until you have rolled it 15 to 20 times. Divide the dough into eight pieces. Roll each piece out into a 6" to 7" circle, flouring both sides of the circle as you roll it. Place the pita breads on lightly floured baking sheets and bake them in the preheated oven until they are lightly browned, about 5 to 9 minutes. Remove them from the oven and immediately wrap them in a very lightly dampened dishcloth. When they are completely cool, remove them from the dishcloth and store them in a plastic bag. Use a serrated knife to cut them in half and open any places where the top and bottom of the pita did not separate.

Nutritional Analysis: (% Daily Value based on a 2000 calorie diet)

	Per batch	Per pita	%D.V.
Calories:	1744	218	11%
Protein (g):	56	7	-
Carbohydrate (g):	311	39	13%
Total fat (g):	30	3.8	6%
Saturated (g):	0	0	0
Cholesterol (mg):	0	0	0
Sodium (mg):	1533	192	8%
Fiber (g):	27	3.4	11%

Serving size: one pita bread
Servings per batch: eight pita breads

Diabetic exchanges per serving: 2¾ starch/bread

Rolls and Buns

Basic Roll or Bun Dough

Ingredients:	**1½ lb. or 1 lb. machine**
Water	⅞ c.
Apple juice concentrate, thawed	¼ c.
Oil	1 tbsp.
Liquid lecithin (or use additional oil)	½ tbsp.
Salt	1 tsp.
Bread flour	3⅛ c.
Active dry yeast	1¾ tsp.

Cycle: Dough cycle. Shape and bake as in the following recipes.

Nutritional Analysis: (% Daily Value based on a 2000 calorie diet)

	Per batch	Per roll	%D.V.
Calories:	1557	104	5%
Protein (g):	43	2.9	-
Carbohydrate (g):	286	19	6%
Total fat (g):	23	1.5	2%
Saturated (g):	0	0	0
Cholesterol (mg):	0	0	0
Sodium (mg):	2031	135	6%
Fiber (g):	0.9	0.06	<1%

Serving size: approximately 1.5 oz.
Servings per batch: 15 for above values

Diabetic exchanges per serving:
    1¼ starch/bread if you make 15 rolls per batch
    1½ starch/bread if you make 12 buns per batch
    1 starch/bread if you make 19 small rolls per batch
Diabetic exchanges per whole recipe: 19 starch/bread

Wheat-free Basic Roll or Bun Dough

Ingredients:	1½ lb. or 1 lb. machine
Water	⅞ c.
Apple juice concentrate, thawed	¼ c.
Oil	1 tbsp.
Liquid lecithin (or may use additional oil)	½ tbsp.
Salt	1 tsp.
White spelt flour	3½ c.
Active dry yeast	1¾ tsp.

Cycle: Dough cycle. Shape and bake as in the following recipes.

Nutritional Analysis: (% Daily Value based on a 2000 calorie diet)

	Per batch	Per roll	%D.V.
Calories:	1708	107	5%
Protein (g):	56	3.5	-
Carbohydrate (g):	314	20	7%
Total fat (g):	24	1.5	2%
Saturated (g):	0	0	0
Cholesterol (mg):	0	0	0
Sodium (mg):	2031	127	5%
Fiber (g):	7	0.4	1%

Serving size: approximately 1.4 oz.
Servings per batch: 16 for above values

Diabetic exchanges per serving:
    1¼ starch/bread if you make 16 rolls per batch
    1¾ starch/bread if you make 12 buns per batch
    1 starch/bread if you make 21 small rolls per batch
Diabetic exchanges per whole recipe: 21 starch/bread

Gluten-free Roll or Bun Dough

Ingredients:	1½ lb. or 1 lb. machine
Water	½ c. + 1 tbsp.
Apple juice concentrate, thawed	¼ c.
Oil	2 tbsp.
Eggs OR egg substitute	3 eggs OR ¾ c.
Salt	1 tsp.
Vitamin C crystals	⅛ tsp.
Guar gum	4 tsp.
Brown rice flour	2 c.
Potato flour	⅓ c.
Tapioca flour	⅓ c.
Active dry yeast	2¼ tsp.

Cycle: Dough cycle. Shape and bake as in the gluten-free recipe on page 140.

Nutritional Analysis: (% Daily Value based on a 2000 calorie diet.)

	Per batch	Per roll	% D.V (roll)	Per bun	% D.V. (bun)
Calories (with eggs):	1891	118	6%	189	9%
(with egg substitute):	1883	118	6%	189	9%
Protein (g):	54	3.4	-	5.4	-
Carbohydrate (g):	325	20	7%	32	10%
Total fat (g) (eggs):	52	3.2	5%	5.2	8%
(with egg substitute):	61	3.8	6%	6.1	9%
Saturated (g) (eggs):	5.1	0.4	2%	0.6	3%
(egg substitute):	0	0	0	0	0
Cholesterol (mg) (eggs):	1029	64	21%	103	34%
(with egg substitute):	0	0	0	0	0
Sodium (mg) (eggs):	2286	143	6%	229	10%
(with egg substitute):	2361	148	6%	236	10%
Fiber (g):	17	1.1	4%	1.7	6%

Serving size: approximately 1.6 oz. for rolls, 2.6 oz. for buns
Servings per batch: 16 rolls or 10 buns for above values
Diabetic exchanges per serving: 1½ starch/bread per roll; 2½ starch/bread per bun
Diabetic exchanges per whole recipe: 24 starch/bread

Bread or Bun Wash

BRUSH THIS ON YOUR BREAD OR BUNS INSTEAD OF EGG WHITE TO MAKE THE CRUST SHINY AND HELP SEEDS OR OTHER TOPPINGS STICK.

¼ c. water
1 tsp. tapioca flour or cornstarch

      Combine the water and starch in a small saucepan, bring them to a boil, reduce the heat, and simmer until the mixture is clear and the consistency of egg white. Or, combine the water and starch in a glass container and microwave them for 45 seconds to 1 minute, stirring every 15 seconds. Allow the wash to cool to lukewarm. Brush it on bread or buns after shaping them and sprinkle with seeds if desired. Allow them to rise and bake as directed in the bread or bun recipe.

Nutritional analysis for the whole batch: 10 calories, 2.5 g. carbohydrate.

Hot Dog Buns

Ingredients:

1 batch of any of the following recipes:
    Basic Roll or Bun Dough, page 126
    Wheat-free Basic Roll or Bun Dough, page 127
    Any 1½ lb. basic bread recipe, pages 61 to 75 or 77 to 78
    Any 1½ lb. whole grain bread recipe, pages 79 to 92,
       99 to 101, 105 to 106, or 108 to 109

Cycle: Dough cycle. When the cycle has finished, divide the dough into 12 pieces. Spray with cooking oil spray or lightly oil three 8″ or 9″ square pans or two 13″ by 9″ pans. Roll the pieces of dough into ropes that are about 7″ to 8″ long, and line them up parallel to each other in the pans. (Put 4 in each square pan or 6 in each rectangular pan.) Allow them to rise for 30 to 45 minutes, or until they have doubled in volume. Bake at 375°F for 15 to 20 minutes, or until browned. Remove them from the pans and put them on racks immediately. Break them apart into individual buns when they are cool.

Nutritional Analysis: Divide the whole batch values for the bread or dough recipe used by 12, or the number of buns you made.
Diabetic exchanges: Divide the total number of exchanges per batch of the recipe you used by the number of buns you made.

Hamburger Buns

Ingredients:

1 batch of any of the following recipes:
  Basic Roll or Bun Dough, page 126
  Wheat-free Basic Roll or Bun Dough, page 127
  Any 1½ lb. basic bread recipe, pages 61 to 75 or 77 to 78
  Any 1½ lb. whole grain bread recipe, pages 79 to 92,
     99 to 101, 105 to 106, or 108 to 109

Cycle: Dough cycle. When the cycle has finished, divide the dough into 12 pieces, or the number necessary to make buns of the size you desire. Spray a baking sheet with cooking oil spray or lightly oil it. Knead the pieces of dough briefly, form them into balls, and put them on the baking sheet. Allow them to rise for 30 to 45 minutes, or until they have doubled in volume. Bake at 375°F for 13 to 18 minutes, or until browned.

Nutritional Analysis: Divide the whole batch values for the bread or dough recipe used by 12 or the number of buns you made.

Diabetic exchanges: Divide the total number of exchanges per batch of the recipe you used by the number of buns you made.

Poppy Seed Rolls or Buns

Ingredients:

1 batch of any of the following recipes:
    Basic Roll or Bun Dough, page 126
    Wheat-free Basic Roll or Bun Dough, page 127
    Any 1½ lb. basic bread recipe, pages 61 to 75 or 77 to 78
    Any 1½ lb. whole grain bread recipe, pages 79 to 92,
        99 to 101, 105 to 106, or 108 to 109
1 slightly beaten egg white or "Bread or Bun Wash," p. 129
1 tbsp. poppy seeds

Cycle: Dough cycle. When the cycle has finished, shape the rolls as directed in any roll or bun recipe in this chapter. Brush them with the egg white or wash, and sprinkle with the poppy seeds. Allow them to rise and bake them as directed in the roll or bun recipe.

Nutritional Analysis: To the whole batch values for the recipe you are using, add 15 calories and 1.5 g. of fat. Divide the whole batch values by the number of buns or rolls you made.

Diabetic exchanges: Divide the total number of exchanges per batch of the recipe you used by the number of buns or rolls you made.

Sesame Seed Rolls or Buns

Prepare as directed in the "Poppy Seed Rolls or Buns" recipe above, except substitute 1 tbsp. sesame seeds for the poppy seeds.

Nutritional Analysis: To the whole batch values for the recipe you are using, add 27 calories, 1 g. protein, and 2.5 g. of fat. Divide the whole batch values by the number of buns or rolls you made.

Diabetic exchanges: Divide the total number of exchanges per batch of the recipe you used by the number of buns or rolls you made.

Onion Rolls or Buns

THESE BUNS ARE GREAT WITH HAMBURGERS.

Ingredients:

1 batch of any of the following recipes:
  Basic Roll or Bun Dough, page 126
  Wheat-free Basic Roll or Bun Dough, page 127
  Any 1½ lb. basic bread recipe, pages 61 to 75 or 77 to 78
  Any 1½ lb. whole grain bread recipe, pages 79 to 92,
    99 to 101, 105 to 106, or 108 to 109
2 tbsp. dried minced onion, divided
2 tbsp. water
1 slightly beaten egg white or "Bread or Bun Wash," p. 129

Cycle: Dough cycle. Add 1 tbsp. of the onion to the dough with the salt when you start the machine. While the cycle is running, soak the remaining 1 tbsp. of onion in the water for 15 minutes; then drain it on paper towel. When the cycle is finished, shape 12 hamburger buns or 16 rolls as on p. 130. Brush them with the egg white or wash and sprinkle them with the drained onion. Allow them to rise for 30 to 45 minutes, or until they have doubled in volume. Bake at 375°F for 13 to 18 minutes, or until browned.

Nutritional Analysis: To the whole batch values for the recipe you are using, add 28 calories and 7 g. carbohydrate. Divide the whole batch values by the number of buns or rolls you made.

Diabetic exchanges: Divide the total number of exchanges per batch of the recipe you used by the number of buns or rolls you made.

Cornmeal Rolls

Ingredients:

1 batch of any of the following recipes:
   White Corn Bread, p. 77
   Wheat-free White Corn Bread, p. 78
   Corny Bread, p. 105
   Wheat-free Corny Bread, p. 106
   Gluten-free Corny Bread, p. 107

Cycle: Dough cycle. When the cycle is finished, knead the dough (except for the gluten-free dough) briefly and form it into 9 to 12 balls. Spray a muffin tin with cooking oil spray or lightly oil it. Place each ball in a muffin cup. For the gluten-free dough, spoon enough dough into each muffin cup to fill it ⅔ full. Allow the rolls to rise until double in volume, 40 to 60 minutes. Bake at 375°F for 15 to 20 minutes, or until brown.

Nutritional Analysis: Divide the whole batch values for the recipe you used by the number of rolls you made.

Diabetic exchanges: Divide the total number of exchanges per batch of the recipe you used by the number of rolls you made.

Cloverleaf Rolls

Ingredients:

1 batch of any of the following recipes:
   Basic Roll or Bun Dough, page 126
   Wheat-free Basic Roll or Bun Dough, page 127
   Any 1½ lb. basic bread recipe, pages 61 to 75 or 77 to 78
   Any 1½ lb. whole grain bread recipe, pages 79 to 92,
      99 to 101, 105 to 106, or 108 to 109

Cycle: Dough cycle. After the cycle is finished, knead the dough briefly on a lightly oiled board. Spray a muffin tin with cooking oil spray or lightly oil it. Shape the dough into 1″ balls. Put three balls into each muffin cup. Allow to rise until double in volume, about 30 to 40 minutes. Bake at 375°F for 15 to 25 minutes, or until lightly browned.

Nutritional Analysis: Divide the whole batch values for the recipe you used by the number of rolls you made.

Diabetic exchanges: Divide the total number of exchanges per batch of the recipe you used by the number of rolls you made.

Fan Tans

Ingredients:

1 batch of any of the following recipes:
   Basic Roll or Bun Dough, page 126
   Wheat-free Basic Roll or Bun Dough, page 127
   Any 1½ lb. basic bread recipe, pages 61 to 75 or 77 to 78
   Any 1½ lb. whole grain bread recipe, pages 79 to 92,
     99 to 101, 105 to 106, or 108 to 109
Cooking oil spray or cooking oil

Cycle: Dough cycle. After the cycle is finished, knead the dough briefly on a lightly oiled board. Spray a muffin tin with cooking oil spray or lightly oil it. Roll the dough out with an oiled rolling pin to ⅛" to ¼" thickness. Cut it into strips 1½" wide. Stack 6 to 7 strips, spraying with cooking oil spray or brushing lightly with oil between layers. Cut the stacks of strips into 1½" segments, and put each into a muffin cup with the cut edges up. Allow to rise until double in volume, about 30 to 40 minutes, and bake at 375°F for 15 to 25 minutes, or until lightly browned.

Nutritional Analysis: Divide the whole batch values for the recipe you used by the number of rolls you made.

Diabetic exchanges: Divide the total number of exchanges per batch of the recipe you used by the number of rolls you made.

Wedgies

Ingredients:

1 batch of any of the following recipes:
  Basic Roll or Bun Dough, page 126
  Wheat-free Basic Roll or Bun Dough, page 127
  Any 1½ lb. basic bread recipe, pages 61 to 75 or 77 to 78
  Any 1½ lb. whole grain bread recipe, pages 79 to 92,
    99 to 101, 105 to 106, or 108 to 109
Cooking oil spray or cooking oil
Cinnamon (optional)

Cycle: Dough cycle. After the cycle is finished, knead the dough briefly on a lightly oiled board. Spray a baking sheet with cooking oil spray or lightly oil it. Roll the dough out with an oiled rolling pin into a circle ⅛″ to ¼″ thick. Cut the circle into quarters, and each quarter into 3 to 4 pieces, so you end up with 12 to 16 triangular pieces of dough. Spray the pieces with cooking oil spray or brush them lightly with oil. If desired, sprinkle them with cinnamon. Roll each wedge up, starting at the wide end. Put them on the baking sheet with the point of the wedge on the bottom of the roll. Allow to rise until double in volume, about 30 to 40 minutes. Bake at 375°F for 15 to 25 minutes, or until lightly browned.

Nutritional Analysis: Divide the whole batch values for the recipe you used by the number of rolls you made.

Diabetic exchanges: Divide the total number of exchanges per batch of the recipe you used by the number of rolls you made.

Parker House Rolls

Ingredients:

1 batch of any of the following recipes:
  Basic Roll or Bun Dough, page 126
  Wheat-free Basic Roll or Bun Dough, page 127
  Any 1½ lb. basic bread recipe, pages 61 to 75 or 77 to 78
  Any 1½ lb. whole grain bread recipe, pages 79 to 92,
    99 to 101, 105 to 106, or 108 to 109

Cycle: Dough cycle. After the cycle is finished, remove the dough from the machine; do not knead it. Spray a baking sheet with cooking oil spray or lightly oil it. Roll the dough out with a lightly oiled rolling pin to ½″ thickness. Cut it into 2½″ to 3″ rounds with a biscuit cutter. Make a deep crease down the center of each round with the handle of a knife. Fold the round over at the crease and press the edges together lightly. Put the rolls on the baking sheet and allow them to rise until double in volume, about 30 to 40 minutes. Bake at 375°F for 15 to 25 minutes, or until lightly browned.

Nutritional Analysis: Divide the whole batch values for the recipe you used by the number of rolls you made.

Diabetic exchanges: Divide the total number of exchanges per batch of the recipe you used by the number of rolls you made.

Pan Rolls

Ingredients:

1 batch of any of the following recipes:
Basic Roll or Bun Dough, page 126
Wheat-free Basic Roll or Bun Dough, page 127
Any 1½ lb. basic bread recipe, pages 61 to 75 or 77 to 78
Any 1½ lb. whole grain bread recipe, pages 79 to 92,
99 to 101, 105 to 106, or 108 to 109
Cooking oil spray or cooking oil

Cycle: Dough cycle. After the cycle is finished, remove the dough from the machine. Knead it briefly on an oiled board. Spray a 9″ x 13″ baking pan with cooking oil spray or lightly oil it. Divide the dough into 15 balls. Spray the balls with cooking oil spray or brush them lightly with oil. Put them into the prepared pan in rows of three. Allow them to rise until double in volume, about 25 to 40 minutes. Bake at 375°F for 25 to 35 minutes, or until lightly browned. Spray them with cooking oil spray or brush them lightly with oil immediately after removing them from the oven.

Nutritional Analysis: Divide the whole batch values for the recipe you used by the number of rolls you made.

Diabetic exchanges: Divide the total number of exchanges per batch of the recipe you used by the number of rolls you made.

Dinner Rolls

Ingredients:

1 batch of any of the following recipes:
    Basic Roll or Bun Dough, page 126
    Wheat-free Basic Roll or Bun Dough, page 127
    Any 1½ lb. basic bread recipe, pages 61 to 75 or 77 to 78
    Any 1½ lb. whole grain bread recipe, pages 79 to 92,
       99 to 101, 105 to 106, or 108 to 109

Cycle: Dough cycle. When the cycle is finished, knead the dough briefly and form it into 12 to 16 balls. Spray a muffin tin with cooking oil spray or lightly oil it. Place each ball in a muffin cup. Allow the rolls to rise until double in volume, 30 to 50 minutes. Bake at 375°F until brown, 15 to 20 minutes.

Nutritional Analysis: Divide the whole batch values for the recipe you used by the number of rolls you made.

Diabetic exchanges: Divide the total number of exchanges per batch of the recipe you used by the number of rolls you made.

Boolots

MY MOTHER ONCE MADE ROLLS FOR A FAMILY CELEBRATION THAT CAME OUT SO LARGE THAT MY GRANDFATHER CALLED THEM "BIG BALLS" IN ITALIAN. THE WORD, WHICH SOUNDED LIKE "BOOLOTS," IS WHAT WE CALL LARGE ROLLS SUCH AS THESE TO THIS DAY.

Ingredients:

1 batch of any of the following recipes:
   Basic Roll or Bun Dough, page 126
   Wheat-free Basic Roll or Bun Dough, page 127
   Any 1½ lb. basic bread recipe, pages 61 to 75 or 77 to 78
   Any 1½ lb. whole grain bread recipe, pages 79 to 92,
      99 to 101, 105 to 106, or 108 to 109

Cycle: Dough cycle. When the cycle is finished, knead the dough briefly and form it into 6 to 8 balls. Spray a "Texas size" muffin tin with cooking oil spray or lightly oil it. Place each ball in a muffin cup. Allow the rolls to rise until double in volume, 40 to 50 minutes. Bake at 375°F until brown, about 20 to 25 minutes.

Nutritional Analysis: Divide the whole batch values for the recipe you used by the number of rolls you made.

Diabetic exchanges: Divide the total number of exchanges per batch of the recipe you used by the number of rolls you made.

Gluten-free or Low-gluten Rolls or Buns

IF YOU MAKE THESE BUNS IN CUSTARD CUPS OR A "TEXAS SIZE" MUFFIN PAN AND SLICE THEM IN HALF HORIZONTALLY, THEY ARE GREAT WITH HAMBURGERS.

Ingredients:

1 batch of any of the following recipes:
    Gluten-free Roll or Bun Dough, p. 128
    Buckwheat Bread, p. 93
    Quinoa Bread, p. 94
    Amaranth Bread, p. 95
    No-egg Brown Rice Bread, p. 96
    Barley Bread, p. 97
    Oat Bread, p. 98
    Gluten-free Corny Bread, p. 107

Cycle: Dough cycle. Spray with cooking oil spray or lightly oil a muffin tin, Texas size muffin tin, or custard cups. When the cycle is finished, put the dough into muffin cups, filling them ⅔ full for rolls. Or, to make hamburger buns, fill them ⅓ to ½ full. Allow them to rise until barely doubled, 20 to 40 minutes. Bake at 375°F for 15 to 25 minutes, or until browned.

Nutritional Analysis: Divide the whole batch values for the recipe you used by the number of rolls or buns you made.

Diabetic exchanges: Divide the total number of exchanges per batch of the recipe you used by the number of rolls or buns you made.

Heart Healthy Crescent Rolls

1 batch of any of the following recipes:
  Basic Roll or Bun Dough, page 126
  Wheat-free Basic Roll or Bun Dough, page 127
  Any 1½ lb. basic bread recipe, pages 61 to 75 or 77 to 78
  Any 1½ lb. whole grain bread recipe, pages 79 to 92,
    99 to 101, 105 to 106, or 108 to 109
Cooking oil spray

Cycle: Dough cycle. After the cycle is finished, knead the dough briefly on a lightly oiled board. Spray a baking sheet with cooking oil spray or lightly oil it. Roll the dough out with an oiled rolling pin into a 12″ to 15″ square about ¼″ thick. Lightly spray the dough with cooking oil spray. Fold it in thirds by folding the right third of the dough over the center third, and then folding the left third over both. Roll the dough to ¼″ thickness again. Turn the dough 90°, spray it with cooking oil, fold it in thirds and roll it to ¼″ thickness again. Repeat the spraying, folding, rolling, and turning process twice more. Roll the dough out into a 12″ square. Cut off the edges and cut the large square into nine 4″ squares. Cut each small square diagonally into a triangle. Starting with one of the short sides, roll up each triangle and put it on the baking sheet with the point under the roll, curving it slightly to form a crescent. Allow it to rise in a warm place for 30 to 40 minutes. Bake at 375°F for 15 to 20 minutes.

Nutritional Analysis: Essentially the same as for the dough used. To get the per serving values, divide the whole batch values for the dough you used by 18.

Diabetic exchanges per serving: Divide the number of starch/bread exchanges for a whole batch of the dough used by 18 to get the exchanges per serving.

Savory Snails

Ingredients:	1½ lb. or 1 lb. machine
Water	⅞ c.
Apple juice concentrate, thawed	¼ c.
Oil	1 tbsp.
Liquid lecithin (or additional oil)	½ tbsp.
Salt	¾ tsp.
Bread flour	3⅛ c.
Active dry yeast	1¾ tsp.
Dried tomato flakes or dried tomatoes cut into ¼″ pieces	⅓ c.
Additional oil	2 tsp.
Grated Romano cheese	¼ to ⅓ c.

Cycle: Dough cycle. Add the ingredients above the dotted line to your machine and start the cycle. About 10 minutes before the last kneading time will finish, add the tomatoes. After the cycle finishes, roll the dough out on a lightly oiled board to a 12″ by 16″ rectangle. Brush with the additional oil and sprinkle with the cheese. Starting with the long side, roll the dough up like a jelly roll and pinch the edge to the roll. Cut it into 15 slices. Put them cut side down into oiled muffin pans and allow to rise until double, about 30 minutes. Bake at 375°F for 15 to 20 minutes, or until nicely browned.

Nutritional Analysis: (% Daily Value based on a 2000 calorie diet)

	Per Batch	Per serving	%D.V.
Calories:	1802	120	6%
Protein (g):	57	3.8	-
Carbohydrate (g):	296	20	7%
Total fat (g):	41	2.7	4%
Saturated (g):	3	0.2	<1%
Cholesterol (mg):	20	1.3	<1%
Sodium (mg):	2051	137	6%
Fiber (g):	3.9	0.3	1%

Serving size: approximately 1.5 oz.; Servings per batch: 15
Diabetic exchanges per serving: 1½ starch/bread

Wheat-free Savory Snails

Ingredients:	1½ lb. or 1 lb. machine
Water	⅞ c.
Apple juice concentrate, thawed	¼ c.
Oil	1 tbsp.
Liquid lecithin (or additional oil)	½ tbsp.
Salt	¾ tsp.
White spelt flour	3⅜ c.
Active dry yeast	1¾ tsp.

- -

Dried tomato flakes or dried tomatoes cut into ¼″ pieces	⅓ c.
Additional oil	2 tsp.
Grated Romano cheese	¼ to ⅓ c.

Cycle: Dough cycle. Add the ingredients above the dotted line to your machine and start the cycle. About 10 minutes before the last kneading time will finish, add the tomatoes. After the cycle finishes, roll the dough out on a lightly oiled board to a 12″ by 16″ rectangle. Brush with the additional oil and sprinkle with the cheese. Starting with the long side, roll the dough up like a jelly roll and pinch the edge to the roll. Cut it into 15 slices. Put them cut side down into oiled muffin pans and allow to rise until double, about 30 minutes. Bake at 375°F for 15 to 20 minutes, or until nicely browned.

Nutritional Analysis: (% Daily Value based on a 2000 calorie diet)

	Per Batch	Per serving	%D.V.
Calories:	1953	130	6%
Protein (g):	70	4.7	-
Carbohydrate (g):	324	22	7%
Total fat (g):	42	2.8	4%
Saturated (g):	3	0.2	<1%
Cholesterol (mg):	20	1.3	<1%
Sodium (mg):	2051	137	6%
Fiber (g):	10	0.7	2%

Serving size: approximately 1.5 oz.; Servings per batch: 15
Diabetic exchanges per serving: 1½ starch/bread

No-Yeast Quick Breads and Cakes

WHEN YOU MAKE NO-YEAST QUICK BREADS OR CAKES IN A BREAD MACHINE, YOU DO NOT ADD ALL OF THE INGREDIENTS AT ONCE, AND YOUR MACHINE MAY REQUIRE SOME ASSISTANCE IN MIXING. FOLLOW THE DIRECTIONS BELOW WHEN MAKING ALL OF THE RECIPES IN THIS CHAPTER.

MIXING DIRECTIONS: Put the flour(s), baking powder, and salt (and baking soda, guar gum, spices, and other dry ingredients, if used) in the bread machine. Press "start" and mix for ½ to 1 minute. (Begin timing AFTER the fast mixing starts if your machine mixes slowly at first.) Add the oil and mix for 1 minute. Add the remaining ingredient(s). If the dough is not evenly distributed in the pan at the end of the mixing time, reach in with a rubber spatula and gently spread it so it covers the bottom of the pan fairly evenly. Scrape down the sides of the pan if necessary.

No-Yeast White Bread

Ingredients:
3 c. all-purpose flour
3 tsp. baking powder
½ tsp. salt
¼ c. oil
1¼ c. water

Cycle: Quick bread or cake, mix as above.

Nutritional Analysis: (% Daily Value based on a 2000 calorie diet)

	Per Loaf	Per serving	%D.V.
Calories:	1680	80	4%
Protein (g):	35	1.7	-
Carbohydrate (g):	251	12	4%
Total fat (g):	56	2.7	4%
Saturated (g):	0	0	0
Cholesterol (mg):	0	0	0
Sodium (mg):	2327	111	5%
Fiber (g):	0.9	0.04	<1%

Serving size: approximately 1.1 oz.; Servings per loaf: 21
Diabetic exchanges per serving: 1 starch/bread

No-Yeast White Spelt Bread

Ingredients:

3 c.   white spelt flour
3 tsp. baking powder
½ tsp. salt
¼ c.   oil
1 c.   water

Cycle: Quick bread or cake, mix as on page 144.

Nutritional Analysis: (% Daily Value based on a 2000 calorie diet)

	Per Loaf	Per serving	%D.V.
Calories:	1725	82	4%
Protein (g):	48	2.3	-
Carbohydrate (g):	252	12	4%
Total fat (g):	59	2.8	4%
Saturated (g):	0	0	0
Cholesterol (mg):	0	0	0
Sodium (mg):	2326	111	5%
Fiber (g):	6	0.3	1%

Serving size: approximately 1.0 oz.
Servings per loaf: 21

Diabetic exchanges per serving: 1 starch/bread

No-Yeast
Whole Wheat Bread

Ingredients:

3 c.   regular (not bread) whole wheat flour
3 tsp. baking powder
½ tsp. salt
¼ c.   oil
1¼ c.   water

Cycle: Cake or quick bread; mix as on p. 144.

Nutritional Analysis: (% Daily Value based on a 2000 calorie diet)

	Per Loaf	Per serving	%D.V.
Calories:	1920	80	4%
Protein (g):	53	2.2	-
Carbohydrate (g):	283	12	4%
Total fat (g):	63	2.6	4%
Saturated (g):	0	0	0
Cholesterol (mg):	0	0	0
Sodium (mg):	2332	97	4%
Fiber (g):	9.3	0.4	1%

Serving size: 1.0 approximately oz.
Servings per loaf: 24

Diabetic exchanges per serving: 1 starch/bread

No-Yeast
Whole Spelt Bread

Ingredients:

3 c.   whole grain spelt flour
3 tsp.   baking powder
½ tsp. salt
¼ c.   oil
1¼ c.   water

Cycle: Quick bread or cake, mix as on page 144.

Nutritional Analysis: (% Daily Value based on a 2000 calorie diet)

	Per Loaf	Per serving	%D.V.
Calories:	1770	80	4%
Protein (g):	48	2.2	-
Carbohydrate (g):	252	11.4	4%
Total fat (g):	62	2.8	4%
Saturated (g):	0	0	0
Cholesterol (mg):	0	0	0
Sodium (mg):	2326	106	4%
Fiber (g):	24	1.1	4%

Serving size: approximately 1.0 oz.
Servings per loaf: 22

Diabetic exchanges per serving: 1 starch/bread

No-Yeast Rye Bread

Ingredients:

3	c.	rye flour
3	tsp.	baking powder
¾	tsp.	salt
2	tsp.	caraway seed (optional)
⅓	c.	oil
1¼	c.	water

Cycle: Quick bread or cake, mix as on page 144.

Nutritional Analysis: (% Daily Value based on a 2000 calorie diet)

	Per Loaf	Per serving	%D.V.
Calories:	1990	83	4%
Protein (g):	43	1.8	-
Carbohydrate (g):	282	12	4%
Total fat (g):	76	3.2	5%
Saturated (g):	0	0	0
Cholesterol (mg):	0	0	0
Sodium (mg):	2824	118	5%
Fiber (g):	48	2	7%

Serving size: approximately 1.0 oz.
Servings per loaf: 24

Diabetic exchanges per serving: 1 starch/bread

No-Yeast White Rye Bread

Ingredients:

3 c.	white rye flour (See "Sources," p. 236.)
3 tsp.	baking powder
¾ tsp.	salt
⅓ c.	oil
1¼ c.	water

Cycle: Quick bread or cake, mix as on page 144.

Nutritional Analysis: (% Daily Value based on a 2000 calorie diet)

	Per Loaf	Per serving	%D.V.
Calories:	1990	83	4%
Protein (g):	43	1.8	-
Carbohydrate (g):	282	12	4%
Total fat (g):	76	3.2	5%
Saturated (g):	0	0	0
Cholesterol (mg):	0	0	0
Sodium (mg):	2824	118	5%
Fiber (g):	1.5	0.06	<1%

Serving size: approximately 1.0 oz.
Servings per loaf: 24

Diabetic exchanges per serving: 1 starch/bread

No-Yeast Barley Bread

Ingredients:

    3 c.   barley flour
    3 tsp. baking powder
    ¾ tsp. salt
    ¼ c.   oil
    1¼ c.   water

Cycle: Quick bread or cake, mix as on page 144.

Nutritional Analysis: (% Daily Value based on a 2000 calorie diet)

	Per Loaf	Per serving	%D.V.
Calories:	1800	82	4%
Protein (g):	30	1.4	-
Carbohydrate (g):	294	13	4%
Total fat (g):	56	2.5	4%
Saturated (g):	0	0	0
Cholesterol (mg):	0	0	0
Sodium (mg):	2832	129	5%
Fiber (g):	1.8	0.08	<1%

Serving size: approximately 1.0 oz.
Servings per loaf: 22

Diabetic exchanges per serving: 1 starch/bread

No-Yeast Kamut Bread

Ingredients:

3	c.	kamut flour
3	tsp.	baking powder
¾	tsp.	salt
⅓	c.	oil
1⅓	c.	water

Cycle: Quick bread or cake, mix as on page 144.

Nutritional Analysis: (% Daily Value based on a 2000 calorie diet)

	Per Loaf	Per serving	%D.V.
Calories:	1960	82	4%
Protein (g):	42	1.8	-
Carbohydrate (g):	282	12	4%
Total fat (g):	74	3.1	5%
Saturated (g):	0	0	0
Cholesterol (mg):	0	0	0
Sodium (mg):	2820	117	5%
Fiber (g):	48	2	7%

Serving size: approximately 1.1 oz.
Servings per loaf: 24

Diabetic exchanges per serving: 1 starch/bread

No-Yeast Gluten-Free Rice Bread

Ingredients:

1⅓ c.	brown rice flour OR white rice flour
⅓ c.	tapioca flour
⅓ c.	potato flour
2¾ tsp.	guar gum
2¾ tsp.	baking powder
¾ tsp.	salt
1 tbsp.	plus 1 tsp. oil
2	extra large eggs OR ½ c. egg substitute
1⅓ c.	water

Cycle: Quick bread or cake, mix as on page 144.

Nutritional Analysis: (% Daily Value based on a 2000 calorie diet)

	Per Loaf	Per serving	%D.V.
Calories (with eggs):	1341	83	4%
(with egg substitute):	1269	79	4%
Protein (g):	30	1.9	-
Carbohydrate (g):	222	14	5%
Total fat (g, with eggs):	17	1.1	2%
(with egg substitute):	23	1.4	2%
Saturated (g, with eggs):	4	0.3	1%
(with egg substitute):	0	0	0
Cholesterol (mg, with eggs):	686	43	10%
(with egg substitute):	0	0	0
Sodium (mg, with eggs):	2884	180	8%
(with egg substitute):	2934	184	8%
Fiber (g, with white rice):	6	0.4	1%
(g, with brown rice):	12	0.8	3%

Serving size: 1.4 approximately oz.
Servings per loaf: 16

Diabetic exchanges per serving: 1 starch/bread

Corn Bread

Ingredients:

1½ c.	all-purpose flour
½ c.	cornmeal
2½ tsp.	baking powder
½ tsp.	salt
2 tbsp.	oil
1	extra large egg OR ¼ c. egg substitute OR ¼ c. water in addition to the amount below
¼ c.	Fruit Sweet™ or honey
⅜ c.	water

Cycle: Quick bread or cake, mix as on page 144.

Nutritional Analysis: (% Daily Value based on a 2000 calorie diet)

	Per Loaf	Per serving	%D.V.
Calories (with egg):	1258	79	4%
(with egg substitute):	1224	77	4%
(with water):	1159	72	4%
Protein (g, with egg or egg substitute):	29	1.8	-
(with water):	21	1.3	-
Carbohydrate (g):	198	12.4	4%
Total fat (g, with egg):	37	2.3	4%
(with egg substitute):	40	2.5	4%
(with water):	30	1.9	3%
Saturated (g, with egg):	2	0.1	<1%
(with egg substitute):	0	0	0
(with water):	0	0	0
Cholesterol (mg, with egg):	343	21	7%
(with egg substitute):	0	0	0
(with water):	0	0	0
Sodium (mg, with egg):	2189	137	6%
(with egg substitute):	2214	138	6%
(with water):	2103	131	5%
Fiber (g):	0.8	0.05	<1%

Serving size: approximately 1.0 oz.
Servings per loaf: 16

Diabetic exchanges per serving: 1 starch/bread

Wheat-free Corn Bread

Ingredients:

1¾ c.	white spelt flour
½ c.	cornmeal
2½ tsp.	baking powder
½ tsp.	salt
2 tbsp.	oil
1	extra large egg OR ¼ c. egg substitute OR ¼ c. water in addition to the amount below
¼ c.	Fruit Sweet™ or honey
⅜ c.	water

Cycle: Quick bread or cake, mix as on page 144.

Nutritional Analysis: (% Daily Value based on a 2000 calorie diet)

	Per Loaf	Per serving	%D.V.
Calories (with egg):	1384	81	4%
(with egg substitute):	1348	79	4%
(with water):	1285	76	4%
Protein (g, with egg or egg substitute):	40	2.4	-
(with water):	32	1.9	-
Carbohydrate (g):	219	13	5%
Total fat (g, with egg):	38	2.2	3%
(with egg substitute):	41	2.4	3%
(with water):	31	1.8	3%
Saturated (g, with egg):	2	0.1	<1%
(with egg substitute):	0	0	0
(with water):	0	0	0
Cholesterol (mg, with egg):	343	20	7%
(with egg substitute):	0	0	0
(with water):	0	0	0
Sodium (mg, with egg):	2189	129	5%
(with egg substitute):	2214	130	5%
(with water):	2103	124	5%
Fiber (g):	3.4	0.2	1%

Serving size: approximately 1.0 oz.
Servings per loaf: 17

Diabetic exchanges per serving: 1 starch/bread

Gluten-free Corn Bread

Ingredients:

1 c.   brown rice flour
½ c.   cornmeal
⅓ c.   tapioca flour
⅓ c.   potato flour
3 tsp. guar gum
3 tsp. baking powder
½ tsp. salt
2 tbsp. oil
2 extra large eggs OR ½ c. egg substitute
¼ c.   Fruit Sweet™ or honey
⅝ c.   water

Cycle: Quick bread or cake, mix as on page 144.

Nutritional Analysis: (% Daily Value based on a 2000 calorie diet)

	Per Loaf	Per serving	%D.V.
Calories (with eggs):	1580	79	4%
(with egg substitute):	1508	76	4%
Protein (g):	35	1.8	-
Carbohydrate (g):	249	12	4%
Total fat (g, with eggs):	45	2	4%
(with egg substitute):	51	3	4%
Saturated (g, with eggs):	4	0.2	<1%
(with egg substitute):	0	0	0
Cholesterol (mg, with eggs):	343	17	6%
(with egg substitute):	0	0	0
Sodium (mg, with eggs):	2492	125	5%
(with egg substitute):	2542	127	5%
Fiber (g):	11	0.6	2%

Serving size: approximately 1.1 oz.
Servings per loaf: 20

Diabetic exchanges per serving: 1 starch/bread

Applesauce Bread

Ingredients:

2 c.	all-purpose flour
1 tsp.	baking powder
½ tsp.	baking soda
½ tsp.	salt (optional)
1 tsp.	cinnamon
¼ c.	oil
½ c.	unsweetened apple juice concentrate, thawed
¾ c.	unsweetened applesauce
½ c.	raisins (optional)

Cycle: Quick bread or cake, mix as on page 144, adding raisins after the liquids are thoroughly mixed in.

Nutritional Analysis: (% Daily Value based on a 2000 calorie diet)

	Per Loaf	Per serving	%D.V.
Calories (with raisins):	1799	90	4%
(without raisins):	1582	79	4%
Protein (g, with raisins):	25	1.1	-
(without raisins):	23	1.1	-
Carbohydrate (g, with raisins):	298	15	5%
(without raisins):	242	12	4%
Total fat (g):	55	2.5	4%
Saturated (g):	0	0	0
Cholesterol (mg):	0	0	0
Sodium (mg, with raisins):	1065	53	2%
(without raisins):	1057	53	2%
Fiber (g, with raisins):	9	0.45	2%
(without raisins):	3	0.15	<1%

Serving size: approximately 1.1 oz.
Servings per loaf: 20

Diabetic exchanges per serving: 1 starch/bread

Wheat-free Applesauce Bread

Ingredients:

2⅜ c.   white spelt flour
1 tsp. baking powder
½ tsp. baking soda
½ tsp. salt (optional)
1 tsp. cinnamon
¼ c.   oil
½ c.   unsweetened apple juice concentrate, thawed
¾ c.   unsweetened applesauce
½ c.   raisins (optional)

Cycle: Quick bread or cake, mix as on page 144, adding raisins after the liquids are thoroughly mixed in.

Nutritional Analysis: (% Daily Value based on a 2000 calorie diet)

	Per Loaf	Per serving	%D.V.
Calories (with raisins):	1985	91	5%
(without raisins):	1768	80	4%
Protein (g, with raisins):	40	1.8	-
(without raisins):	38	1.7	-
Carbohydrate (g, with raisins):	331	15	5%
(without raisins):	275	12	4%
Total fat (g):	58	2.6	4%
Saturated (g):	0	0	0
Cholesterol (mg):	0	0	0
Sodium (mg, with raisins):	1966	89	4%
(without raisins):	1958	89	4%
Fiber (g, with raisins):	14	0.7	2%
(without raisins):	8	0.4	1%

Serving size: approximately 1.0 oz.
Servings per loaf: 22

Diabetic exchanges per serving: 1 starch/bread

Quinoa Applesauce Bread

Ingredients:

2½ c.	quinoa flour
¾ c.	tapioca flour
3 tsp.	baking powder
½ tsp.	baking soda
2 tsp.	cinnamon
¼ c.	oil
¾ c.	unsweetened apple juice concentrate, thawed
¾ c.	unsweetened applesauce
½ c.	raisins (optional)

Cycle: Quick bread or cake, mix as on page 144, adding raisins after the liquids are thoroughly mixed in.

Nutritional Analysis: (% Daily Value based on a 2000 calorie diet)

	Per Loaf	Per serving	%D.V.
Calories (with raisins):	2507	86	4%
(without raisins):	2290	79	4%
Protein (g, with raisins):	35	1.2	-
(without raisins):	33	1.1	-
Carbohydrate (g, with raisins):	453	15.6	5%
(without raisins):	397	13.7	5%
Total fat (g):	65	2.2	3%
Saturated (g):	0	0	0
Cholesterol (mg):	0	0	0
Sodium (mg, with raisins):	1864	64	3%
(without raisins):	1856	64	3%
Fiber (g, with raisins):	21	0.7	2%
(without raisins):	15	0.5	2%

Serving size: approximately 1.0 oz.
Servings per loaf: 29

Diabetic exchanges per serving: 1 starch/bread

Date Nut Bread

Ingredients:

2 c.	all purpose flour
½ c.	date sugar
3 tsp.	baking powder
⅜ c.	oil
¾ c.	apple juice concentrate, thawed
¾ c.	chopped dates
¾ c.	chopped walnuts or other nuts

Cycle: Quick bread or cake, mix as on page 144, adding dates and nuts after the liquids are thoroughly mixed in. If the sides of this bread seem to be getting too brown before the baking time is up, test the center of the cake by inserting a toothpick into it. If it comes out dry, stop the cycle early and remove the bread.

Nutritional Analysis: (% Daily Value based on a 2000 calorie diet)

	Per Loaf	Per serving	%D.V.
Calories:	3150	175	9%
Protein (g):	45	2.5	-
Carbohydrate (g):	477	26.5	9%
Total fat (g):	97	5.4	8%
Saturated (g):	0	0	0
Cholesterol (mg):	0	0	0
Sodium (mg):	1379	77	3%
Fiber (g):	17	0.9	3%

Serving size: approximately 1.4 oz.
Servings per loaf: 18

Diabetic exchanges per serving: 1 starch/bread + 1 fruit + 1 fat

Spelt Date Nut Bread

Ingredients:

2¼ c.   whole spelt or white spelt flour
½ c.   date sugar
3 tsp.   baking powder
⅜ c.   oil
¾ c.   apple juice concentrate, thawed
¾ c.   chopped dates
¾ c.   chopped walnuts or other nuts

Cycle: Quick bread or cake, mix as on page 144, adding dates and nuts after the liquids are thoroughly mixed in. If the sides of this bread seem to be getting too brown before the baking time is up, test the center of the cake by inserting a toothpick into it. If it comes out dry, stop the cycle early and remove the bread.

Nutritional Analysis: (% Daily Value based on a 2000 calorie diet)

	Per Loaf	Per serving	%D.V.
Calories:	3274	182	9%
Protein (g):	58	3.2	-
Carbohydrate (g):	499	28	9%
Total fat (g):	99	5.5	8%
Saturated (g):	0	0	0
Cholesterol (mg):	0	0	0
Sodium (mg):	1379	77	3%
Fiber (g, whole spelt):	31	1.7	6%
(g, white spelt):	17	0.9	3%

Serving size: approximately 1.4oz.
Servings per loaf: 18

Diabetic exchanges per serving: 1 starch/bread + 1 fruit + 1 fat

Barley Date Nut Bread

Ingredients:

2 c.	barley flour
½ c.	date sugar
3 tsp.	baking powder
⅜ c.	oil
¾ c.	apple juice concentrate, thawed
¾ c.	chopped dates
¾ c.	chopped walnuts or other nuts

Cycle: Quick bread or cake, mix as on page 144, adding dates and nuts after the liquids are thoroughly mixed in. If the sides of this bread seem to be getting too brown before the baking time is up, test the center of the cake by inserting a toothpick into it. If it comes out dry, stop the cycle early and remove the bread.

Nutritional Analysis: (% Daily Value based on a 2000 calorie diet)

	Per Loaf	Per serving	%D.V.
Calories:	3220	179	9%
Protein (g):	42	2.3	-
Carbohydrate (g):	506	28	9%
Total fat (g):	97	5.4	8%
Saturated (g):	0	0	0
Cholesterol (mg):	0	0	0
Sodium (mg):	1383	77	3%
Fiber (g):	14	0.8	3%

Serving size: approximately 1.4 oz.
Servings per loaf: 18

Diabetic exchanges per serving: 1 starch/bread + 1 fruit + 1 fat

Golden Fruit Bread

Ingredients:

   3 c. kamut flour

   3 tsp. baking powder

   ¼ tsp. salt

   ⅓ c. oil

   1⅓ c. apple juice concentrate, thawed

   ⅓ c. dried blueberries, raisins, dried apricots cut into small pieces, or small pieces of the dried fruit of your choice

Cycle: Quick bread or cake. Mix as on page 144, adding the dried fruit after the apple juice is thoroughly mixed in. Watch the bread as the cycle nears completion, and if the sides of the loaf are getting too brown, test the bread for doneness by inserting a toothpick into the center of the bread. If the toothpick comes out dry, stop the cycle early and remove the bread from the machine.

Nutritional Analysis: (% Daily Value based on a 2000 calorie diet)

	Per Loaf	Per serving	%D.V.
Calories:	2697	108	5%
Protein (g):	44	1.8	-
Carbohydrate (g):	468	19	6%
Total fat (g):	74	3	5%
Saturated (g):	0	0	0
Cholesterol (mg):	0	0	0
Sodium (mg):	1917	77	3%
Fiber (g):	52	2.1	7%

Serving size: approximately 1.25 oz.;   Servings per loaf: 25

Diabetic exchanges per serving: 1 starch/bread + ½ fruit

Banana Spice Cake

Ingredients:

2 c.	all purpose flour
½ c.	date sugar
2½ tsp.	baking powder
½ tsp.	salt
1½ tsp.	cinnamon
¼ tsp.	cloves
¼ tsp.	allspice
¼ c.	oil
2 c.	pureed or thoroughly mashed bananas
½ tsp.	vanilla (optional)

Cycle: Quick bread or cake, mix as on page 144.

Nutritional Analysis: (% Daily Value based on a 2000 calorie diet)

	Per Cake	Per serving	%D.V.
Calories:	2576	143	7%
Protein (g):	34	1.9	-
Carbohydrate (g):	504	28	9%
Total fat (g):	57	32	5%
Saturated (g):	0	0	0
Cholesterol (mg):	0	0	0
Sodium (mg):	2104	117	5%
Fiber (g):	13	0.7	2%

Serving size: approximately 1.5 oz.
Servings per cake: 18

Diabetic exchanges per serving: 1 starch/bread + 1 fruit

Wheat-free Banana Spice Cake

Ingredients:

2 c.	barley flour
½ c.	date sugar
3 tsp.	baking powder
1½ tsp.	cinnamon
¼ tsp.	cloves
¼ tsp.	allspice
¼ c.	oil
2¼ c.	pureed or thoroughly mashed bananas
½ tsp.	vanilla (optional)

Cycle: Quick bread or cake, mix as on page 144. If the sides of this cake seem to be getting too brown before the baking time is up, test the center of the cake by inserting a toothpick into it. If it comes out dry, stop the cycle early and remove the cake.

Nutritional Analysis: (% Daily Value based on a 2000 calorie diet)

	Per Cake	Per serving	%D.V.
Calories:	2780	139	7%
Protein (g):	32	1.6	-
Carbohydrate (g):	566	28	9%
Total fat (g):	57	2.9	4%
Saturated (g):	0	0	0
Cholesterol (mg):	0	0	0
Sodium (mg):	1328	66	3%
Fiber (g):	14	0.7	2%

Serving size: approximately 1.5 oz.
Servings per cake: 20

Diabetic exchanges per serving: 1 starch/bread + 1 fruit

Gluten-free Banana Spice Cake

Ingredients:

2¼ c.   brown rice flour
½ c.   tapioca flour
½ c.   date sugar
3 tsp.   baking powder
1½ tsp. cinnamon
¼ tsp.   cloves
¼ tsp.   allspice
¼ c.   oil
2¼ c.   pureed or thoroughly mashed bananas
½ tsp.   vanilla (optional)

Cycle: Quick bread or cake, mix as on page 144. If the sides of this cake seem to be getting too brown before the baking time is up, test the center of the cake by inserting a toothpick into it. If it comes out dry, stop the cycle early and remove the cake.

Nutritional Analysis: (% Daily Value based on a 2000 calorie diet)

	Per Cake	Per serving	%D.V.
Calories:	3215	140	7%
Protein (g):	39	1.7	-
Carbohydrate (g):	660	29	10%
Total fat (g):	59	2.6	4%
Saturated (g):	0	0	0
Cholesterol (mg):	0	0	0
Sodium (mg):	1321	57	2%
Fiber (g):	23	1	3%

Serving size: approximately 1.5 oz.
Servings per cake: 23

Diabetic exchanges per serving: 1 starch/bread + 1 fruit

Chocolate Cake

Ingredients:

2⅓ c.   all purpose flour
⅓ c.   cocoa
3 tsp.   baking powder
¼ tsp.   salt
¼ c.   oil
1¼ c.   apple juice concentrate, thawed

Cycle: Quick bread or cake, mix as on page 144. If the sides of this cake seem to be getting too brown before the baking time is up, test the center of the cake by inserting a toothpick into it. If it comes out dry, stop the cycle early and remove the cake.

Nutritional Analysis: (% Daily Value based on a 2000 calorie diet)

	Per Cake	Per serving	%D.V.
Calories:	2059	108	5%
Protein (g):	32	1.7	-
Carbohydrate (g):	338	18	6%
Total fat (g):	61	2.7	4%
Saturated (g):	2	0.1	<1%
Cholesterol (mg):	0	0	0
Sodium (mg):	1912	101	4%
Fiber (g):	2.7	0.1	<1%

Serving size: approximately 1.2 oz.
Servings per cake: 19

Diabetic exchanges per serving: 1 starch/bread + ½ fruit

Wheat-free Chocolate Cake

Ingredients:

2¾ c.   white spelt flour
⅓ c.   cocoa
3 tsp. baking powder
¼ tsp. salt
¼ c.   oil
1¼ c.   apple juice concentrate, thawed

Cycle: Quick bread or cake, mix as on page 144. If the sides of this cake seem to be getting too brown before the baking time is up, test the center of the cake by inserting a toothpick into it. If it comes out dry, stop the cycle early and remove the cake.

Nutritional Analysis: (% Daily Value based on a 2000 calorie diet)

	Per Cake	Per serving	%D.V.
Calories:	2267	108	5%
Protein (g):	49	2.3	-
Carbohydrate (g):	374	18	6%
Total fat (g):	66	3	5%
Saturated (g):	0	0	0
Cholesterol (mg):	0	0	0
Sodium (mg):	1912	101	4%
Fiber (g):	24	1.1	4%

Serving size: approximately 1.2 oz.
Servings per cake: 21

Diabetic exchanges per serving: 1 starch/bread + ½ fruit

Gluten-free Chocolate Cake

Ingredients:

1¼ c.   brown rice OR white rice flour
⅓ c.   tapioca flour
⅓ c.   potato flour
⅓ c.   cocoa
2¾ tsp. guar gum
2½ tsp. baking powder + ½ tsp. baking soda with
         Fruit Sweet™ OR 3 tsp. baking powder with honey
¼ tsp. salt
 2 tbsp. oil
 2 extra large eggs OR ½ c. egg substitute
¾ c.   Fruit Sweet™ or honey
½ c.   water

Cycle: Quick bread or cake, mix as on page 144. If the sides of this cake seem to be getting too brown before the baking time is up, test the center of the cake by inserting a toothpick into it. If it comes out dry, stop the cycle early and remove the bread.

Nutritional Analysis: (% Daily Value based on a 2000 calorie diet)

	Per Cake	Per serving	%D.V.
Calories (with eggs):	2197	110	5%
(with egg substitute):	2125	106	5%
Protein (g):	39	1.9	-
Carbohydrate (g):	398	20	7%
Total fat (g, with eggs):	48	2.4	4%
(with egg substitute):	54	2.7	4%
Saturated (g, with eggs):	4	0.2	<1%
(with egg substitute):	2	0.1	<1%
Cholesterol (mg, with eggs):	686	34	11%
(with egg substitute):	0	0	0
Sodium (mg, with eggs):	2034	102	4%
(with egg substitute):	2082	104	4%
Fiber (g, brown rice flour):	13	0.7	2%
(g, white rice flour):	8	0.4	1%

Serving size: approximately 1.25 oz.; Servings per cake: 20

Diabetic exchanges per serving: 1 starch/bread + ½ fruit

Extra Nutrition Carrot Cake

Ingredients:

2⅛	c.	whole wheat flour
1½	tsp.	baking soda
1	tsp.	cinnamon
¼	tsp.	cloves
3	tbsp.	oil
⅔	c.	pineapple juice concentrate
⅔	c.	water
1	c.	shredded carrots
½	c.	raisins

Cycle: Quick bread or cake, mix as on page 144, adding the carrots and raisins after the liquids are thoroughly mixed in.

Nutritional Analysis: (% Daily Value based on a 2000 calorie diet)

	Per Cake	Per serving	%D.V.
Calories:	1974	110	6%
Protein (g):	44	2.4	-
Carbohydrate (g):	356	20	7%
Total fat (g):	47	2.6	4%
Saturated (g):	0	0	0
Cholesterol (mg):	0	0	0
Sodium (mg):	1556	86	4%
Fiber (g):	15	0.8	3%

Serving size: approximately 1.4 oz.
Servings per cake: 18

Diabetic exchanges per serving: 1 starch/bread + ½ fruit

Wheat-free Extra Nutrition Carrot Cake

Ingredients:

2⅛ c.   rye flour
1½ tsp. baking soda
1 tsp.   cinnamon
¼ tsp.   cloves
3 tbsp. oil
⅔ c.   pineapple juice concentrate
⅔ c.   water
1 c.   shredded carrots
½ c.   raisins

Cycle: Quick bread or cake, mix as on page 144, adding the carrots and raisins after the liquids are thoroughly mixed in.

Nutritional Analysis: (% Daily Value based on a 2000 calorie diet)

	Per Cake	Per serving	%D.V.
Calories:	1910	112	6%
Protein (g):	37	2.2	-
Carbohydrate (g):	355	21	7%
Total fat (g):	44	2.6	4%
Saturated (g):	0	0	0
Cholesterol (mg):	0	0	0
Sodium (mg):	1551	91	4%
Fiber (g):	18	1	3%

Serving size: approximately 1.4 oz.
Servings per cake: 17

Diabetic exchanges per serving: 1 starch/bread + ½ fruit

Extra Nutrition Gingerbread

Ingredients:

  2 c.   whole wheat flour
  2 tsp. baking powder
  1 tsp. cinnamon
  ½ tsp. ginger
  3 tbsp. oil
  ½ c.   molasses
  ½ c.   water

Cycle: Quick bread or cake, mix as on page 144.

Nutritional Analysis: (% Daily Value based on a 2000 calorie diet)

	Per Cake	Per serving	%D.V.
Calories:	1620	81	4%
Protein (g):	35	1.8	-
Carbohydrate (g):	279	14	5%
Total fat (g):	47	2.3	4%
Saturated (g):	0	0	0
Cholesterol (mg):	0	0	0
Sodium (mg):	1032	52	2%
Fiber (g):	6	0.3	1%

Serving size: approximately 0.9 oz.
Servings per cake: 20

Diabetic exchanges per serving: 1 starch/bread

Wheat-free Extra Nutrition Gingerbread

Ingredients:

2⅜ c.	whole spelt flour
2 tsp.	baking powder
1 tsp.	cinnamon
½ tsp.	ginger
3 tbsp.	oil
½ c.	molasses
½ c.	water

Cycle: Quick bread or cake, mix as on page 144.

Nutritional Analysis: (% Daily Value based on a 2000 calorie diet)

	Per Cake	Per serving	%D.V.
Calories:	1741	79	4%
Protein (g):	38	1.7	-
Carbohydrate (g):	290	13	4%
Total fat (g):	47	2.1	3%
Saturated (g):	0	0	0
Cholesterol (mg):	0	0	0
Sodium (mg):	1029	47	2%
Fiber (g):	19	0.9	3%

Serving size: approximately 0.9 oz.
Servings per cake: 22

Diabetic exchanges per serving: 1 starch/bread

Creamy Cake Topping

THIS SUGAR-FREE TOPPING IS GREAT ON CHOCOLATE CAKE, CARROT CAKE, OR GINGERBREAD, PAGES 166 TO 172.

Ingredients:

½ c.   unsalted cashews, macadamias, or shelled pine nuts
1 tbsp. tapioca flour
2 tsp.   cocoa (optional - use if you want chocolate topping)
⅓ c.   Fruit Sweet™ or liquid Fruit Source™
½ tsp.   vanilla (optional)

Put the nuts and tapioca flour in a blender or food processor and process until the nuts are finely ground. Add the optional cocoa, if desired, and process for a few seconds. With the blender or processor running, slowly add the sweetener. Add the vanilla and process a few more seconds.

Nutritional Analysis: To the whole batch values for the cake you are using this topping on add 613 calories, 13 g. protein, 67 g. carbohydrate, 32 g. fat, 10 mg. sodium, and 6 g. fiber

Diabetic exchanges per whole batch: 5 fruit + 7 fat

Heart Healthy Date Frosting

THIS FAT-FREE, SUGAR-FREE FROSTING IS GOOD ON BANANA SPICE
CAKE OR DATE NUT BREAD, PAGES 163 TO 165 AND 159 TO 161.

Ingredients:

⅜ c. + 1 tbsp. water

1 tbsp. all purpose flour OR 1 tbsp. white spelt flour OR
      1 tbsp. barley flour OR 1 tbsp. + 1 tsp. rice flour

⅔ c. date sugar

Combine the flour and water in a small saucepan. Bring them
to a boil, reduce the heat, and simmer, stirring often, until the
mixture is thick. Remove from the heat. Press the date sugar
through a sieve to remove lumps. Add it to the flour mixture
and beat until smooth. Frost the cake immediately before the
frosting has time to cool.

Nutritional Analysis: To the whole batch values for the cake you are using this topping on add 428 calories, 107 g. carbohydrate, and 10 g. fiber.

Diabetic exchanges per whole batch: 7 fruit

Bread Based Main Dishes & Snacks

Heart-Healthy Burgers

Ingredients:

1 lb.	ground turkey (be sure this does not contain skin)
½ lb.	ground buffalo
1 c.	cooked grain of any kind or combination
1 c.	cooked vegetables, any kind or combination (peas, beans, and carrots are good)
1 tsp.	salt, or to taste (optional)
	Hamburger buns, p. 130

Briefly puree the grains and vegetables in a food processor or blender. (They do not have to be liquified; a few chunks remaining in the burgers are nice.) Combine the puree with the turkey, buffalo, and salt and form the mixture into 10 patties. Broil 5 to 8 minutes on each side and serve with the buns. These patties freeze well.

Nutritional Analysis: (Values based on using brown rice for the grain and ⅓ c. each of peas, carrots, and green beans. The values include the burgers only and not the buns. % Daily Value based on a 2000 calorie diet.)

	Per batch	Per serving	%D.V.
Calories:	1396	140	7%
Protein (g):	189	19	-
Carbohydrate (g):	65	6	2%
Total fat (g):	37	3.7	6%
Saturated (g):	13	1.3	6%
Cholesterol (mg):	497	50	17%
Sodium (mg):	2588	259	11%
Fiber (g):	2.8	0.3	1%

Serving size: approximately 3 oz.;   Servings per batch: 10

Diabetic exchanges per serving: 2 lean meat plus ½ starch/bread

Dumpling Pie

Filling Ingredients:

½ c.   chopped celery
¼ c.   chopped onion OR additional chopped celery
2 tbsp. oil
3 tbsp. all purpose flour OR white spelt flour
¼ tsp. dry sweet basil OR 1 tsp. fresh chopped sweet basil
¼ tsp. pepper
1½ c.   chicken or turkey broth
1½ c.   peas, frozen or fresh
2 c.   cubed cooked turkey or chicken

To make the filling, saute the celery and onion in the 2 tbsp. oil until they begin to brown. Add the 3 tbsp. flour and stir and cook 1 minute. Add the seasonings and broth; bring the mixture to a boil and cook a few minutes until it is thickened. Stir in the peas and chicken or turkey. Put the filling into a 2½ to 3-qt. casserole dish. Preheat the oven to 400°F.

Topping Ingredients:

1 c.   all purpose OR white spelt flour
1 tsp. baking powder
¼ tsp. salt
¼ tsp. dry sweet basil OR 1 tsp. fresh chopped sweet basil
2 tbsp. oil
⅓ c.   water

To make the topping, put the 1 c. flour, baking powder, salt, and basil into your bread machine pan. Set the cycle to "mix" if your machine has that cycle; otherwise, the first few minutes of any cycle will work fine. Start the machine and let it mix for ½ to 1 minute. (If it mixes very slowly at first, begin timing when the fast, continuous mixing begins.) Add the oil and allow it to mix another minute. Add the water and allow the machine to mix for about 2 minutes, or until about 30 seconds after the dough has become a cohesive ball around the bread machine blade. Stop the machine.

Remove the dough from the machine and drop heaping teaspoonfuls of it onto the filling mixture in the casserole. Bake for 30 to 35 minutes, or until the dumplings are lightly browned.

Nutritional Analysis: (% Daily Value based on a 2000 calorie diet)

	Per batch	Per serving	%D.V.
Calories:	1672	279	14%
Protein (g):	113	19	-
Carbohydrate (g):	140	23	8%
Total fat (g):	56	9	14%
Saturated (g):	5	0.8	4%
Cholesterol (mg):	215	36	12%
Sodium (mg):	1989	331	14%
Fiber (g):	10.5	1.8	6%

Serving size: 1/6 of the batch
Servings per batch: 6

Diabetic exchanges per serving: 2 starch/bread + 2 lean meat

Tamale Pie

Filling Ingredients:

¼ c.		chopped bell pepper (about ½ pepper)
½		small onion, chopped (optional)
1 tbsp.		oil
1 15-oz.		can tomatoes
1 tsp.		chili powder
1 4-oz.		can sliced mushrooms, drained
1 14-oz.		can black beans, drained
1 c.		cubed cooked turkey or chicken

To make the filling, saute the pepper and onion in the oil until they begin to brown. Coarsely chop the tomatoes and add them and their juice to the saucepan. Stir in the chili powder, mushrooms, beans, and chicken or turkey and bring the mixture to a boil. Pour it into a 2½ to 3-qt. casserole dish. Preheat the oven to 350°F.

Topping Ingredients:

½ c.	all purpose OR white spelt flour
½ c.	cornmeal
2 tsp.	baking powder
¼ tsp.	salt
2 tbsp.	oil
½ c.	water

To make the topping, put the flour, cornmeal, baking powder, and salt into your bread machine pan. Set the cycle to "mix" if your machine has that cycle; otherwise, the first few minutes of any cycle will work fine. Start the machine and let it mix for ½ to 1 minute. (If it mixes very slowly at first, begin timing when the fast, continuous mixing begins.) Add the oil and allow it to mix another minute. Add the water and allow the machine to mix for another 1 to 2 minutes. Stop the machine.

Spread the batter over the filling mixture in the casserole dish. Bake for 30 to 35 minutes, or until the topping begins to brown.

Nutritional Analysis: (% Daily Value based on a 2000 calorie diet)

	Per batch	Per serving	%D.V.
Calories:	1583	264	13%
Protein (g):	88	15	-
Carbohydrate (g):	189	31	11%
Total fat (g):	51	8.5	13%
Saturated (g):	2	0.3	1%
Cholesterol (mg):	107	18	6%
Sodium (mg):	4019	670	28%
Fiber (g):	32	5	18%

Serving size: 1/6 of the batch
Servings per batch: 6

Diabetic exchanges per serving: 2 starch/bread + 2 lean meat

Heart Healthy Pizza

Dough ingredients:

¾ c.	water
2½ tbsp.	apple juice concentrate, thawed
1 tbsp	oil
½ tsp.	salt
2¼ c.	bread flour
1¼ tsp.	active dry yeast

Sauce ingredients (for 2 pizzas - freeze half for future use):

1 6-oz.	can tomato paste
1 8-oz.	can tomato sauce
½ c.	water
1 tsp.	dry oregano OR 1 tbsp. chopped fresh oregano
½ tsp.	dry thyme OR 1 tsp. chopped fresh thyme
½ tsp.	dry sweet basil OR 1 tsp. chopped fresh sweet basil

Topping ingredients:

2 to 3 oz.	low fat or part-skim mozzarella cheese
2 tbsp.	grated Romano cheese
½ c.	chopped vegetables of your choice - green peppers, mushrooms, etc.
2 oz.	cooked lean ground meat (optional)

Start the dough in your bread machine using the dough cycle. Combine the sauce ingredients in a saucepan, bring them to a boil, reduce the heat, and simmer them for 30 to 40 minutes, stirring occasionally. Grate the cheese and chop the vegetables. Preheat your oven to 400°F. When the dough cycle is finished, remove the dough from the bread machine and stretch it out in a lightly oiled 12″ pizza pan. Spread it with half of the sauce and sprinkle it with the toppings. If you prefer "thick crust" pizza, allow the pizza to rise for 20 to 30 minutes. For a thinner crust, bake it as soon as you finish making it. Bake for 25 to 30 minutes, or until the edge of the pizza is brown.

Nutritional Analysis: (% Daily Value based on a 2000 calorie diet)

	Per whole Pizza	Per serving	%D.V.
Calories:	1845	205	10%
Protein (g):	66	7	-
Carbohydrate (g):	246	27	9%
Total fat (g):	60	7	10%
Saturated (g):	10	1	5%
Cholesterol (mg):	61	7	2%
Sodium (mg):	3306	367	15%
Fiber (g):	3	0.3	1%

Serving size: 1/9 pizza
Servings per batch: 9

Diabetic exchanges per serving: 2 starch/bread + ½ medium fat meat + ½ vegetable

Wheat-free Heart-Healthy Pizza

Dough ingredients:

⅔ c.   water
2½ tbsp. apple juice concentrate, thawed
1 tbsp oil
½ tsp.   salt
2¼ c.   white spelt flour
1¾ tsp. active dry yeast

Sauce and topping ingredients: same as for "Heart Healthy Pizza," page 180

Put the dough ingredients into your bread machine and start the dough cycle. Make, top, and bake the pizza as in "Heart Healthy Pizza," page 180.

Nutritional Analysis: (% Daily Value based on a 2000 calorie diet)

	Per whole Pizza	Per serving	%D.V.
Calories:	1884	209	10%
Protein (g):	77	8.5	-
Carbohydrate (g):	251	28	9%
Total fat (g):	62	7	11%
Saturated (g):	10	1	5%
Cholesterol (mg):	61	7	2%
Sodium (mg):	3357	373	16%
Fiber (g):	6.4	0.7	2%

Serving size: 1/9 pizza
Servings per batch: 9

Diabetic exchanges per serving: 2 starch/bread + ½ medium fat meat + ½ vegetable

Gluten-free Pizza

Ingredients:

1 1-lb. batch of "Gluten-free Rice Potato Bread" dough, p. 76

Sauce and topping ingredients from "Heart Healthy Pizza," p. 180

Put the bread ingredients into your bread machine and start the dough cycle. Make, top, and bake the pizza as for "Heart Healthy Pizza," p. 180.

Nutritional Analysis: (% Daily Value based on a 2000 calorie diet)

	Per whole Pizza	Per serving	%D.V.
Calories (with eggs):	1923	192	10%
(egg substitute):	1917	192	10%
Protein (g):	79	8	-
Carbohydrate (g):	247	25	8%
Total fat (g, eggs):	57	5.7	9%
(egg substitute):	64	6.4	10%
Saturated (g, eggs):	14	1.4	6%
(egg substitute):	10	1.0	5%
Cholesterol (mg, eggs):	747	75	25%
(egg substitute):	61	6	2%
Sodium (mg, eggs):	4574	457	19%
(egg substitute):	5146	515	21%
Fiber (g):	13	1.3	4%

Serving size: 1/10 pizza
Servings per pizza: 10

Diabetic exchanges per serving: 2 starch/bread + ½ medium fat meat + ½ vegetable

Easy Vegetarian Burgers

Ingredients:

1 8-oz. can tomato sauce
¾ c.   textured vegetable protein (dry flakes)
¾ c.   oatmeal, uncooked
1 extra large egg OR ¼ c. egg substitute
½ tsp. salt
¼ tsp. pepper
1 tbsp. chopped fresh onion OR 1 tsp. dry minced
        onion flakes (optional)
        Hamburger buns, p. 130

Bring the tomato sauce to a boil in a saucepan. Stir in the textured vegetable protein, remove the pan from the heat, and allow it to stand for 5 to 10 minutes, or until the liquid is all absorbed. Mix in the rest of the ingredients (except the buns). Form the mixture into 6 patties. Cook them in a lightly oiled or non-stick skillet until they brown lightly on both sides. These burgers freeze well, both before and after cooking.

Nutritional Analysis: (These values include the burgers only and not the buns. % Daily Value based on a 2000 calorie diet)

	Per batch	Per serving	%D.V.
Calories (with eggs):	608	101	5%
(egg substitute):	572	95	5%
Protein (g):	69	11.5	-
Carbohydrate (g):	68	11	4%
Total fat (g, eggs):	11	1.8	3%
(egg substitute):	14	2.3	3%
Saturated (g, eggs):	2	0.3	1%
(egg substitute):	0	0	0
Cholesterol (mg, eggs):	343	57	19%
(egg substitute):	0	0	0
Sodium (mg, eggs):	1998	333	14%
(egg substitute):	2333	389	16%
Fiber (g):	0.8	0.1	<1%

Serving size: one burger; Servings per batch: 6

Diabetic exchanges per serving: 1 lean meat + ½ starch/bread

Calzones

Ingredients:

1 batch of dough from any of the following recipes:
  Any 1½ lb. basic bread recipe, pages 61 to 71
  Any 1½ lb. whole grain bread recipe, pages 79 to 81, or
      90 to 92, or 108 to 109
¾ c. low fat or part skim ricotta cheese
¼ c. grated Romano cheese
¼ lb. low fat or part skim mozzarella cheese,
    coarsely grated
½ to ¾ c. pizza sauce, about ¼ of the batch of sauce made for
    "Heart Healthy Pizza," p. 180

Cycle: Dough cycle, using the bread ingredients only. When the cycle is finished, divide the dough into 8 to 10 pieces and roll each piece out into a 6" to 7" circle on a lightly floured board. Mix the cheeses and put the mixture on the circles of dough, evenly dividing it between the circles of dough. Top each cheese portion with about 1 tbsp. of sauce. Moisten the edges of the circles with a small amount of water and fold the circles in half over the filling, crimping the edges together. Prick the tops of the calzones with a sharp knife. Transfer them to a lightly oiled baking sheet and allow to rise in a warm place for 15 to 20 minutes. Preheat the oven to 400°F. Bake the calzones for 20 to 25 minutes, or until brown.

Nutritional Analysis: (These values are for the filling only and must be added to ¹⁄₁₀ of the whole batch values for the bread recipe you use. % Daily Value based on a 2000 calorie diet)

	Per batch	Per serving	%D.V.
Calories:	941	94	5%
Protein (g):	80	8	-
Carbohydrate (g):	26	2.6	1%
Total fat (g):	53	5.3	8%
Saturated (g):	30	3	14%
Cholesterol (mg):	209	21	7%
Sodium (mg):	3825	383	16%
Fiber (g):	0	0	<1%

Serving size: one calzone; Servings per batch: 10

Diabetic exchanges per serving: 1 medium fat meat + ⅓ vegetable + approximately 2 starch/bread. (Divide the number of starch/bread exchanges per batch of the bread recipe you used by 10.)

Vegetable Calzones

Ingredients:

1 batch of dough from any of the following recipes:
    Any 1½ lb. basic bread recipe, pages 61 to 71
    Any 1½ lb. whole grain bread recipe, pages 79 to 81, or
           90 to 92, or 108 to 109
2 to 3 cups cooked vegetables, any kind or combination,
    such as beans, carrots, small pieces of broccoli, sauteed
    mushrooms or onions
¼ lb. low fat or part skim mozzarella cheese, low fat cheddar
    cheese, or low fat monterey jack cheese, coarsely grated

Cycle: Dough cycle, using the bread ingredients only. When the cycle is finished, divide the dough into 8 to 10 pieces and roll each piece out into a 6" to 7" circle on a lightly floured board. Divide the vegetables evenly between the circles of dough. Top each with cheese. Moisten the edges of the circles with a small amount of water and fold the circles in half over the filling, crimping the edges together. Prick the tops of the calzones with a sharp knife. Transfer them to a lightly oiled baking sheet and allow to rise in a warm place for 15 to 20 minutes. Preheat the oven to 400°F. Bake for 20 to 25 minutes, or until brown.

Nutritional Analysis: (These values are for the filling only and must be added to ¹⁄₁₀ of the whole batch values for the bread recipe you used. The values are based on using 1 c. carrots or beans, 1 c. broccoli, and 1 c. mushrooms or onions. % Daily Value based on a 2000 calorie diet)

	Per batch	Per serving	%D.V.
Calories:	515	52	3%
Protein (g):	46	4.6	-
Carbohydrate (g):	34	3.4	1%
Total fat (g):	25	2.5	4%
Saturated (g):	12	1.2	5%
Cholesterol (mg):	80	8	3%
Sodium (mg):	1022	102	4%
Fiber (g):	15	1.5	5%

Serving size: one calzone;   Servings per batch: 10

Diabetic exchanges per serving: ½ medium fat meat + ½ vegetable + approximately 2 starch/bread. (Divide the number of starch/bread exchanges per batch of the bread recipe you used by 10.)

Mexican Strata

Ingredients:

3 to 4 slices of bread from any recipe in this book
1 lb.   fresh or frozen corn
2 lbs. zucchini or crookneck squash, thinly sliced
1-4 oz. can diced green chilies, drained
4 oz.   low fat monterey jack cheese, coarsely grated
3 eggs OR ¾ c. egg substitute
1¾ c.   skim milk
½ tsp. salt
⅛ tsp. pepper

Cut and piece the bread to fit the bottom of an 11" by 7" baking dish. Spread the corn on top of the bread. Cover it with the squash. Spread the chilies on top of the squash. Sprinkle the whole dish with grated cheese. Beat together the remaining ingredients and pour them over the whole dish. Refrigerate overnight or a few hours if desired. Bake, uncovered, at 375°F for 30 to 40 minutes, or until it puffs up and begins to brown.

Nutritional Analysis: (% Daily Value based on a 2000 calorie diet)

	Per batch	Per serving	%D.V.
Calories (with eggs):	1153	192	10%
(egg substitute):	1145	191	10%
Protein (g):	81	13.5	-
Carbohydrate (g):	120	20	7%
Total fat (g, eggs):	52	8.7	13%
(egg substitute):	61	10.1	16%
Saturated (g, eggs):	17	3	14%
(egg substitute):	12	2	9%
Cholesterol (mg, eggs):	1109	185	61%
(egg substitute):	80	13	4%
Sodium (mg, eggs):	2624	437	18%
(egg substitute):	2699	450	19%
Fiber (g):	14	2.3	8%

Serving size: 1/6 batch
Servings per batch: 6

Diabetic exchanges per serving: 1½ starch/bread + 1½ low fat meat

Breadsticks

Ingredients:

1 batch of dough from any of these recipes:
   Any 1½ lb. basic bread recipe, pages 61 to 64 or 69 to 71
   Any 1½ lb. whole grain bread recipe, pages 79 to 91, 99 to
      101, 105 to 106, or 108 to 109
   1 lb. batch of Kamut Bread, page 92
1 lightly beaten egg white OR 1 batch of
      "Bread or Bun Wash," p. 129

Optional for seeded breadsticks:
   ½ c. sesame seeds OR ¼ c. poppy seeds

Cycle: Dough cycle. When the cycle is finished, remove the dough from the machine and divide it into 18 or more pieces. On a lightly floured board, roll each piece into a 10″ long rope. Place them on a lightly oiled baking sheet and brush them with the egg white or wash. Allow them to rise in a warm place for 30 minutes. Preheat your oven and bake at 375°F for 15 to 25 minutes, or until they are brown. Remove them from the baking sheet immediately and cool them on a wire rack.

For seeded breadsticks, after rolling the dough into ropes, brush the breadsticks with the egg white or wash while they are still on the work surface. Then roll them in the seeds and transfer them to the baking sheet. Allow to rise and bake as above.

Nutritional Analysis: For plain breadsticks, divide the whole batch values for the bread recipe you used by the number of breadsticks you made. For sesame seed breadsticks, add 322 calories, 9.6 g. protein, 15 g. carbohydrate, 27 g. fat, 6 mg. sodium, and 11 g. fiber to the whole batch bread values; then divide by the number of breadsticks made. For poppy seed breadsticks, add 190 calories, 6 g. protein, 8 g. carbohydrate, 16 g. fat, 7 mg. sodium, and 3 g. fiber to the whole batch bread values; then divide by the number of breadsticks made.

Diabetic exchanges per serving: Divide the number of starch/bread exchanges in a whole batch of the bread recipe you used by the number of breadsticks made.

Pretzels

Ingredients:

1 batch of dough from any of these recipes:
    Any 1½ lb. basic bread recipe, pages 61 to 64 or 69 to 71
    Any 1½ lb. whole grain bread recipe, pages 79 to 91, 99 to
        101, 105 to 106, or 108 to 109
    1 lb. batch of Kamut Bread, page 92
1 lightly beaten egg white or 1 batch of
    "Bread or Bun Wash," p. 129
1½ tsp. coarse kosher salt

Cycle: Dough cycle. When the cycle is finished, remove the dough from the machine and divide it into 25 to 30 pieces. (One way to do this is to the roll the dough out ½" thick on a lightly floured board and cut it into strips.) Lightly flour your hands and work surface, and roll each piece into a 12" to 15" long rope. Twist each rope into a pretzel or open knot shape. Place them on a lightly oiled baking sheet and brush them with the egg white or wash. Sprinkle them with the salt. Allow them to rise in a warm place for 30 minutes. Preheat your oven and bake at 350°F for 20 to 25 minutes, or until they are lightly brown. Remove them from the baking sheet immediately and cool them on a wire rack.

Nutritional Analysis: To the whole batch values for the bread recipe you used add 3000 mg. sodium. Divide by the number of pretzels you made to get the values per pretzel.

Diabetic exchanges per serving: Divide the number of starch/bread exchanges in a whole batch of the bread recipe you used by the number of pretzels made.

Special Occasion Breads & Desserts

Cinnamon Raisin Bread

Ingredients:	1½ lb. loaf	1 lb. loaf
Water	1⅛ c.	¾ c.
Oil	1½ tbsp.	1 tbsp.
Liquid lecithin (or may use additional oil)	½ tbsp.	1 tsp.
Date sugar	⅓ c.	¼ c.
Salt	1 tsp.	¾ tsp.
Cinnamon	1½ tsp.	1 tsp.
Bread flour	3 c.	2 c.
Active dry yeast	1¾ tsp.	1¼ tsp.
Raisins	½ c.	⅓ c.

Cycle: Raisin bread or basic yeast bread. Put all of the ingredients except the raisins into your machine and start the cycle. When the "beep" of the raisin bread cycle sounds, or 5 to 8 minutes before the end of the last kneading time, add the raisins to the machine. When the bread is done, drizzle with any sweet roll glaze, p. 223 to 224, if desired.

Nutritional Analysis: (% Daily Value based on a 2000 calorie diet)

	Large Loaf	Small Loaf	Per serving	%D.V.
Calories:	1873	1249	78	4%
Protein (g):	43	29	1.8	-
Carbohydrate (g):	357	238	15	5%
Total fat (g):	31	21	1.3	2%
Saturated (g):	0	0	0	0
Cholesterol (mg):	0	0	0	0
Sodium (mg):	2023	1349	84	4%
Fiber (g):	12	8	0.5	2%

Serving size: approximately 1.0 oz.; Servings per large loaf: 24
Servings per small loaf: 16

Diabetic exchanges per serving: 1 starch/bread

Wheat-free Cinnamon Raisin Bread

Ingredients:	1½ lb. loaf	1 lb. loaf
Water	1¼ c.	¾ c. + 1 tbsp.
Oil	1½ tbsp.	1 tbsp.
Liquid lecithin (or may use additional oil)	½ tbsp.	1 tsp.
Date sugar	⅓ c.	¼ c.
Salt	1 tsp.	¾ tsp.
Cinnamon	1½ tsp.	1 tsp.
White spelt flour	3¾ c.	2⅝ c.
Active dry yeast	2¼ tsp.	1¼ tsp.
Raisins	½ c.	⅓ c.

Cycle: Raisin bread or basic yeast bread. Put all of the ingredients except the raisins into your machine and start the cycle. When the "beep" of the raisin bread cycle sounds, or 5 to 8 minutes before the end of the last kneading time, add the raisins to the machine. When the bread is done, drizzle with any sweet roll glaze, p. 223 to 224, if desired.

Nutritional Analysis: (% Daily Value based on a 2000 calorie diet)

	Large Loaf	Small Loaf	Per serving	%D.V.
Calories:	2235	1490	80	4%
Protein (g):	65	43	2.3	-
Carbohydrate (g):	426	284	15	5%
Total fat (g):	34	23	1.2	2%
Saturated (g):	0	0	0	0
Cholesterol (mg):	0	0	0	0
Sodium (mg):	2026	1351	72	3%
Fiber (g):	19	13	0.7	2%

Serving size: approximately 1.0 oz.; Servings per large loaf: 28
Servings per small loaf: 19

Diabetic exchanges per serving: 1 starch/bread

Gluten-free Cinnamon Raisin Bread

Ingredients:	1½ lb. loaf		1 lb. loaf	
Water	¾	c.	½	c.
Oil	2	tbsp.	1½	tbsp.
Eggs OR egg substitute	3	eggs OR ¾ c.	2	eggs OR ½ c.
Salt	1	tsp.	¾	tsp.
Vitamin C crystals	⅛	tsp.	Scant ⅛	tsp.
Guar gum	4	tsp.	3	tsp.
Cinnamon	1½	tsp.	1	tsp.
Brown rice flour	2	c.	1⅓	c.
Potato flour	⅓	c.	¼	c.
Tapioca flour	⅓	c.	¼	c.
Date sugar	⅓	c.	¼	c.
Active dry yeast	2¼	tsp.	1½	tsp.
Raisins	½	c.	⅓	c.

Cycle: Raisin bread or basic yeast bread. Put all of the ingredients except the raisins into your machine and start the cycle. When the "beep" of the raisin bread cycle sounds, or 5 to 8 minutes before the end of the last kneading time, add the raisins to the machine. After the last kneading is finished, spread the dough evenly in the pan. When the bread is done, drizzle with any sweet roll glaze, p. 223 to 224, if desired.

Nutritional Analysis: (% Daily Value based on a 2000 calorie diet)

	Large Loaf	Small Loaf	Per serving	%D.V.
Calories (with eggs):	1980	1320	79	4%
(egg substitute):	1972	1315	79	4%
Protein (g):	54	36	2.2	-
Carbohydrate (g):	348	232	9	3%
Total fat (g, eggs):	52	35	2.1	3%
(egg substitute):	61	41	2.4	4%
Saturated (g, eggs):	5	3	0.2	<1%
(egg substitute):	0	0	0	0
Cholesterol (mg, eggs):	1029	686	41	14%
(egg substitute):	0	0	0	0
Sodium (mg, eggs):	2269	1513	91	4%
(egg substitute):	2344	1563	94	4%
Fiber (g):	22	15	0.9	3%

Serving size: approximately 1.1 oz.; Servings per large loaf: 25
Servings per small loaf: 17

Diabetic exchanges per serving: 1 starch/bread

Challah

Ingredients:	1½ lb. or 1 lb. machine
Water	1 c.
Fruit Sweet™ or honey	¼ c.
Oil	1 tbsp.
Liquid lecithin (or may use additional oil)	½ tbsp.
Salt	1 tsp.
Optional saffron OR yellow food coloring	A small pinch Several drops
Bread flour	3¼ c.
Active dry yeast	2¼ tsp.

1 slightly beaten egg white OR "Bread or Bun Wash," p. 129
A very small pinch of saffron
    OR 1 to 2 drops of yellow food coloring
Sesame seeds, about 2 tsp.

Cycle: Dough cycle, using the ingredients above the dotted line. When the cycle is finished, remove the dough from the machine. Divide it into 4 parts and roll each into a 20″ long rope. Lay them side by side on an oiled baking sheet. Braid them by starting with the rope on the right side; bring it over its immediate neighbor, under the next rope, and over the last rope. Repeat the process over and over, starting from the right, until the loaf is all braided. Brush with the egg white or glaze mixed with saffron or food coloring and sprinkle with the sesame seeds. Allow to rise until double, 30 to 40 minutes, and bake at 375°F for 25 to 30 minutes, or until brown.

Nutritional Analysis: (% Daily Value based on a 2000 calorie diet)

	Per Loaf	Per serving	%D.V.
Calories:	1620	81	4%
Protein (g):	45	2.3	-
Carbohydrate (g):	300	15	5%
Total fat (g):	24	1.2	2%
Saturated (g):	0	0	0
Cholesterol (mg):	0	0	0
Sodium (mg):	2016	101	4%
Fiber (g):	5	0.3	1%

Serving size: approximately 1.1 oz.; Servings per loaf: 20

Diabetic exchanges per serving: 1 starch/bread

Wheat-free Challah

Ingredients: **1½ lb. or 1 lb. machine**
Water   1   c.
Fruit Sweet™ or honey   ¼   c.
Oil   1   tbsp.
Liquid lecithin (or may   ½   tbsp.
  use additional oil)
Salt   1   tsp.
Optional saffron   A small pinch
  OR yellow food coloring   Several drops
White spelt flour   3¾   c.
Active dry yeast   2¼   tsp.

- -

1 slightly beaten egg white OR "Bread or Bun Wash," p. 129
A very small pinch of saffron
  OR 1 to 2 drops of yellow food coloring
Sesame seeds, about 2 tsp.

Cycle: Dough cycle, using the ingredients above the dotted line.
When the cycle is finished, remove the dough from the
machine. Divide it into 4 parts and roll each into a 20" long
rope. Lay them side by side on an oiled baking sheet. Braid
them by starting with the rope on the right side; bring it over
its immediate neighbor, under the next rope, and over the last
rope. Repeat the process over and over, starting from the right,
until the loaf is all braided. Brush with the egg white or glaze
mixed with saffron or food coloring and sprinkle with the
sesame seeds. Allow to rise until double, 30 to 40 minutes, and
bake at 375°F for 25 to 30 minutes, or until brown.

Nutritional Analysis: (% Daily Value based on a 2000 calorie diet)

	Per Loaf	Per serving	%D.V.
Calories:	1876	82	4%
Protein (g):	63	2.7	-
Carbohydrate (g):	348	15	5%
Total fat (g):	27	1.2	2%
Saturated (g):	0	0	0
Cholesterol (mg):	0	0	0
Sodium (mg):	2016	88	4%
Fiber (g):	11	0.5	2%

Serving size: approximately 1.0 oz.; Servings per loaf: 23

Diabetic exchanges per serving: 1 starch/bread

Cranberry Orange Bread

THIS IS GREAT FOR THANKSGIVING.

Use the recipe for Cinnamon Raisin Bread," p. 190, "Wheat-free Cinnamon Raisin Bread," p. 191, or "Gluten-free Cinnamon Raisin Bread," p. 192, except substitute an equal amount of dried cranberries (craisins) for the raisins. For the cinnamon, substitute 1 tbsp. grated orange peel in the 1½ lb. loaf or 2 tsp. grated orange peel in the 1 lb. loaf. If desired, drizzle with "Orange Glaze," p. 224.

Nutritional Analysis: Essentially the same as for the recipe used. From the 1½ lb. loaf whole batch values for the recipe you used, subtract 42 calories, 1 g. protein, 10 g. carbohydrate, and 3 g. fiber. The per serving values and % Daily Value are essentially the same as those in the recipe used.

Serving size and number of servings per loaf: Same as in the recipe used

Diabetic exchanges per serving: 1 starch/bread

Blueberry Lemon Bread

Use the recipe for Cinnamon Raisin Bread," p. 190, "Wheat-free Cinnamon Raisin Bread," p. 191, or "Gluten-free Cinnamon Raisin Bread," p. 192, except substitute an equal amount of dried blueberries for the raisins. For the cinnamon, substitute 1 tbsp. grated lemon peel in the 1½ lb. loaf or 2 tsp. grated lemon peel in the 1 lb. loaf. If desired, drizzle with "Lemon Glaze," p. 223.

Nutritional Analysis: Essentially the same as for the recipe used

Serving size and number of servings per loaf: Same as in the recipe used

Diabetic exchanges per serving: 1 starch/bread

NOTE about adding dried, candied, or glace fruits to the following recipes: Dried fruits can be added in ⅓ c. to 1 c. amounts to any recipe without making any adjustments. Glace or candied fruits contain a variable amount of liquid. Try to drain them thoroughly before you add them, and watch the dough, because you will probably also need to add an additional 2 to 4 tbsp. flour to maintain the right consistency.

Sugarplum Bread

Ingredients:	1½ lb. or 1 lb. machine
Water	¾ c.
Fruit Sweet™ or honey	¼ c.*
Oil	1½ tbsp.
Liquid lecithin (or may use additional oil)	½ tbsp.
Salt	½ tsp.
Nutmeg	½ tsp.
Bread flour	2½ c.
Active dry yeast	2¼ tsp.
Raisins	½ c.
Dried fruit (small pieces of cherries, pineapple, papaya) OR glace or candied fruit* (cherries, pineapple)	½ c.

Cycle: Dough cycle, using the ingredients above the dotted line. Add the raisins and fruit 5 to 10 minutes before the last kneading finishes. After the cycle ends, remove the dough and shape it into a ball on an oiled baking sheet. Allow it to rise in a warm place until double, about 50 to 70 minutes. Bake at 350°F for 35 to 50 minutes, covering it with foil if it browns too quickly.

*If you use glace or candied fruit rather than dried fruit, reduce the amount of sweetener to 3 tbsp. You will probably also have to add 2 to 4 tbsp. flour with the fruit to maintain the right consistency of the dough. The bread will not be sugar-free.

Nutritional Analysis: (% Daily Value based on a 2000 calorie diet)

	Per Loaf	Per serving	%D.V.
Calories:	1821	79	4%
Protein (g):	40	1.7	-
Carbohydrate (g):	354	15	5%
Total fat (g):	34	1.5	2%
Saturated (g):	0	0	0
Cholesterol (mg):	0	0	0
Sodium (mg):	2034	88	4%
Fiber (g):	25	1.1	4%

Serving size: approximately 1.1 oz.; Servings per loaf: 23
Diabetic exchanges per serving: 1 starch/bread

Wheat-free Sugarplum Bread

Ingredients:	1½ lb. or 1 lb. machine
Water	¾ c.
Fruit Sweet™ or honey	¼ c.*
Oil	1½ tbsp.
Liquid lecithin (or may use additional oil)	½ tbsp.
Salt	½ tsp.
Nutmeg	½ tsp.
White spelt flour	3 c.
Active dry yeast	2¼ tsp.
- - - - - - - - - - - - - - - - - - -	- - - - - - - - - -
Raisins	½ c.
Dried fruit (small pieces of cherries, pineapple, papaya) OR glace or candied fruit* (cherries, pineapple)	½ c.

Cycle: Dough cycle, using the ingredients above the dotted line. Add the raisins and fruit 5 to 10 minutes before the last kneading finishes. After the cycle ends, remove the dough and shape it into a ball on an oiled baking sheet. Allow it to rise in a warm place until double, about 50 to 70 minutes. Bake at 350°F for 35 to 50 minutes, covering it with foil if it browns too quickly.

*If you use glace or candied fruit rather than dried fruit, reduce the amount of sweetener to 3 tbsp. You will probably also have to add 2 to 4 tbsp. flour with the fruit to maintain the right consistency of the dough. The bread will not be sugar-free.

Nutritional Analysis: (% Daily Value based on a 2000 calorie diet)

	Per Loaf	Per serving	%D.V.
Calories:	2066	79	4%
Protein (g):	56	2.1	-
Carbohydrate (g):	401	15	5%
Total fat (g):	34	1.3	2%
Saturated (g):	0	0	0
Cholesterol (mg):	0	0	0
Sodium (mg):	2034	78	3%
Fiber (g):	23	0.9	3%

Serving size: approximately 1.0 oz.; Servings per loaf: 26

Diabetic exchanges per serving: 1 starch/bread

Mexican Holiday Bread

Ingredients: 1½ lb. or 1 lb. machine
Water   ¾   c.
Fruit Sweet™ or honey*   ¼   c.
Oil   1½ tbsp.
Liquid lecithin (or may   ½   tbsp.
  use additional oil)
Salt   ¾   tsp.
Grated orange peel   1½ tsp. (packed)
Bread flour   2½ c.
Active dry yeast   1½ tsp.
- -
Dry sweet cherries OR glace   ½   c.
  or candied cherries*, halved
Any glaze, p. 223 to 224, and additional cherries (optional)

Cycle: Dough cycle, using the ingredients above the dotted line. Add the cherries 5 to 10 minutes before the last kneading finishes. After the cycle ends, remove the dough and shape it into a ring on an oiled baking sheet. Allow it to rise in a warm place until double, about 30 to 45 minutes. Bake at 375°F for 25 to 40 minutes, covering it with foil if it browns too quickly. When cool, glaze and top the loaf with additional cherries, if desired.

*If you use glace or candied fruit rather than dried fruit, reduce the amount of sweetener to 3 tbsp. You will probably also have to add 2 to 4 tbsp. flour with the fruit to maintain the right consistency of the dough. The bread will not be sugar-free.

Nutritional Analysis: (% Daily Value based on a 2000 calorie diet)

	Per Loaf	Per serving	%D.V.
Calories:	1653	79	4%
Protein (g):	39	1.9	-
Carbohydrate (g):	307	15	5%
Total fat (g):	31	1.5	2%
Saturated (g):	0	0	0
Cholesterol (mg):	0	0	0
Sodium (mg):	1520	72	3%
Fiber (g):	13	0.6	2%

Serving size: approximately 1.1 oz.; Servings per loaf: 21
Diabetic exchanges per serving: 1 starch/bread

Wheat-free
Mexican Holiday Bread

Ingredients:	1½ lb. or 1 lb. machine
Water	¾ c.
Fruit Sweet™ or honey*	¼ c.
Oil	1½ tbsp.
Liquid lecithin (or may use additional oil)	½ tbsp.
Salt	¾ tsp.
Grated orange peel	1½ tsp. (packed)
White spelt flour	3 c.
Active dry yeast	2 tsp.

- -

Dry sweet cherries OR glace   ½ c.
or candied cherries*, halved
Any glaze, p. 223 to 224, and additional cherries (optional)

Cycle: Dough cycle, using the ingredients above the dotted line. Add the cherries 5 to 10 minutes before the last kneading finishes. After the cycle ends, remove the dough and shape it into a ring on an oiled baking sheet. Allow it to rise in a warm place until double, about 30 to 45 minutes. Bake at 375°F for 25 to 40 minutes, covering it with foil if it browns too quickly. When cool, glaze and top the loaf with additional cherries, if desired.

*If you use glace or candied fruit rather than dried fruit, reduce the amount of sweetener to 3 tbsp. You will probably also have to add 2 to 4 tbsp. flour with the fruit to maintain the right consistency of the dough. The bread will not be sugar-free.

Nutritional Analysis: (% Daily Value based on a 2000 calorie diet)

	Per Loaf	Per serving	%D.V.
Calories:	1903	79	4%
Protein (g):	56	2.3	-
Carbohydrate (g):	355	15	5%
Total fat (g):	34	1.4	2%
Saturated (g):	0	0	0
Cholesterol (mg):	0	0	0
Sodium (mg):	1522	63	3%
Fiber (g):	12	0.5	2%

Serving size: approximately 1.0 oz.; Servings per loaf: 24
Diabetic exchanges per serving: 1 starch/bread

Pannetone

Ingredients:	1½ lb. or 1 lb. machine	
Water	⅞	c.
Fruit Sweet™ or honey	3	tbsp.
Oil	1½	tbsp.
Liquid lecithin (or may use additional oil)	½	tbsp.
Salt	¾	tsp.
Yellow food coloring (optional)	3 to 4	drops
Bread flour	3	c.
Active dry yeast	2¼	tsp.
Golden raisins	¼	c.
Currants	¼	c.
Chopped citron (optional)	3	tbsp.

Cycle: Dough cycle, using the ingredients above the dotted line. Add the raisins, currants, and citron 5 to 10 minutes before the last kneading finishes. After the cycle ends, remove the dough, knead it briefly on a lightly floured board, and shape it into a ball. Place it on an oiled baking sheet or in an oiled and wax paper-lined round casserole dish. Allow it to rise in a warm place until double, about 30 to 45 minutes. Bake at 375°F for 40 to 50 minutes. Remove it from the baking sheet or casserole immediately.

Nutritional Analysis: (% Daily Value based on a 2000 calorie diet)

	Per Loaf	Per serving	%D.V.
Calories:	1927	80	4%
Protein (g):	44	1.8	-
Carbohydrate (g):	371	15	5%
Total fat (g):	30	1.3	2%
Saturated (g):	0	0	0
Cholesterol (mg):	0	0	0
Sodium (mg):	1543	64	3%
Fiber (g):	10	0.4	1%

Serving size: approximately 1.0 oz.; Servings per loaf: 24

Diabetic exchanges per serving: 1 starch/bread

Wheat-free Pannetone

Ingredients:	1½ lb. or 1 lb. machine
Water	¾ c. + 1 tbsp.
Fruit Sweet™ or honey	3 tbsp.
Oil	1½ tbsp.
Liquid lecithin (or may use additional oil)	½ tbsp.
Salt	¾ tsp.
Yellow food coloring (optional)	3 to 4 drops
White spelt flour	3 c.
Active dry yeast	2¼ tsp.
Golden raisins	¼ c.
Currants	¼ c.
Chopped citron (optional)	3 tbsp.

Cycle: Dough cycle, using the ingredients above the dotted line. Add the raisins, currants, and citron 5 to 10 minutes before the last kneading finishes. After the cycle ends, remove the dough, knead it briefly on a lightly floured board, and shape it into a ball. Place it on an oiled baking sheet or in an oiled and wax paper-lined round casserole dish. Allow it to rise in a warm place until double, about 30 to 45 minutes. Bake at 375°F for 40 to 50 minutes. Remove it from the baking sheet or casserole immediately.

Nutritional Analysis: (% Daily Value based on a 2000 calorie diet)

	Per Loaf	Per serving	%D.V.
Calories:	1972	79	4%
Protein (g):	53	2.1	-
Carbohydrate (g):	376	15	5%
Total fat (g):	33	1.3	2%
Saturated (g):	0	0	0
Cholesterol (mg):	0	0	0
Sodium (mg):	1543	62	3%
Fiber (g):	15	0.6	2%

Serving size: approximately 1.0 oz.; Servings per loaf: 25

Diabetic exchanges per serving: 1 starch/bread

Hawaiian Bread

Ingredients:	**1½ lb. or 1 lb. machine**	
Coconut milk	½	c.
Pineapple juice concentrate, thawed	¼	c.
Pureed or thoroughly mashed banana	½ (about 1	c. medium)
Oil	2	tsp.
Liquid lecithin (or may use additional oil)	1	tsp.
Salt	½	tsp.
Bread flour	2⅔	c.
Active dry yeast	1¾	tsp.
Dry diced pineapple	⅓	c.
Unsweetened coconut (optional)	¼	c.
"Pineapple Glaze," p. 224 (optional)		

Cycle: Dough cycle, using the ingredients above the dotted line. Add the pineapple and coconut 5 to 10 minutes before the last kneading finishes. After the cycle ends, remove the dough, knead it briefly on a lightly floured board, and shape it into a ball. Place it in an oiled pie dish. Allow it to rise in a warm place until double, about 40 to 60 minutes. Bake at 375°F for 30 to 40 minutes. Cover it with foil for the last 20 minutes of baking to prevent excessive browning. Remove it from the pie dish immediately. When cool, drizzle with the glaze, if desired.

Nutritional Analysis: (% Daily Value based on a 2000 calorie diet)

	Per Loaf	Per serving	%D.V.
Calories:	2002	80	4%
Protein (g):	45	1.8	-
Carbohydrate (g):	349	14	5%
Total fat (g):	47	1.9	3%
Saturated (g):	27	1.1	5%
Cholesterol (mg):	0	0	0
Sodium (mg):	1102	44	2%
Fiber (g):	11	0.4	1%

Serving size: approximately 1.0 oz.
Servings per loaf: 25

Diabetic exchanges per serving: 1 starch/bread

Wheat-free Hawaiian Bread

Ingredients:	1½ lb. or 1 lb. machine	
Coconut milk	½	c.
Pineapple juice concentrate, thawed	¼	c.
Pureed or thoroughly mashed banana	½ (about 1	c. medium)
Oil	2	tsp.
Liquid lecithin (or may use additional oil)	1	tsp.
Salt	½	tsp.
White spelt flour	3	c.
Active dry yeast	2	tsp.
Dry diced pineapple	⅓	c.
Unsweetened coconut (optional)	¼	c.
"Pineapple Glaze," p. 224 (optional)		

Cycle: Dough cycle, using the ingredients above the dotted line. Add the pineapple and coconut 5 to 10 minutes before the last kneading finishes. After the cycle ends, remove the dough, knead it briefly on a lightly floured board, and shape it into a ball. Place it in an oiled pie dish. Allow it to rise in a warm place until double, about 40 to 60 minutes. Bake at 375°F for 30 to 40 minutes. Cover it with foil for the last 20 minutes of baking to prevent excessive browning. Remove it from the pie dish immediately. When cool, drizzle with the glaze, if desired.

Nutritional Analysis: (% Daily Value based on a 2000 calorie diet)

	Per Loaf	Per serving	%D.V.
Calories:	2182	81	4%
Protein (g):	58	2.1	-
Carbohydrate (g):	383	14	5%
Total fat (g):	50	1.9	3%
Saturated (g):	27	1.0	5%
Cholesterol (mg):	0	0	0
Sodium (mg):	1101	41	2%
Fiber (g):	16	0.6	2%

Serving size: approximately 0.9 oz.; Servings per loaf: 27

Diabetic exchanges per serving: 1 starch/bread

Jam Crescents or Ring

Ingredients:

1 batch of any sweet roll dough, pages 217 to 221
⅓ to ½ c. all-fruit (sugar-free) jam
⅓ c. chopped walnuts or other nuts
2 tsp. cinnamon
Any sweet roll glaze, pages 223 to 224 (optional)

Cycle: Dough cycle, using dough ingredients only. When the cycle finishes, knead the dough briefly on a lightly floured board. Oil a baking sheet. To make two crescents, divide the dough in half and roll each out to a 8″ by 8″ square. Spread with the jam and sprinkle with the nuts and cinnamon, leaving about ¾″ of dough plain around the edges. Roll up jelly-roll fashion, crimp the outer edge to the roll, and squeeze the ends together. Lay the rolls on the baking sheet with the seam down and curve them into crescent shapes. Using a sharp knife, make 7 cuts from the outer edge of the crescent to within about 1½″ of the inner edge. Turn the slices on their sides, all facing the same direction.

To make a ring, roll the dough out to a 12″ by 12″ square. Spread all but a 1″ margin on one edge of the square with jam, and sprinkle it with the nuts and cinnamon. Roll the square up jelly-roll fashion, beginning with the edge opposite the edge without jam. Lay the roll seam side down on the baking sheet. Using a sharp knife, make 11 cuts through one side of the roll to within about 1½″ of the other side of the roll. Form the roll into a circle with the cut edge on the outside. Turn the slices on their sides, all facing the same direction.

Allow the crescents or ring to rise in a warm place until double, about 40 to 50 minutes. Bake at 375°F until nicely browned, about 18 to 25 minutes for the crescents and 20 to 30 minutes for the ring. Remove from the baking sheet immediately and drizzle with glaze if desired.

Nutritional Analysis: To the whole batch values for the dough recipe you used, add 528 calories, 10 g. protein, 72 g. carbohydrate, 22 g. fat, 1.5 g. saturated fat, 12 mg. sodium, and 4 g. fiber. Divide by the number of servings you cut your crescents or ring into to get the per serving values.

Diabetic exchanges per serving: To the whole batch values for the dough recipe you used, add 4½ fruit and 5½ fat exchanges. Divide by the number of servings you cut your crescents or ring into to get the number of exchanges per serving.

Streusel Coffee Cake

Ingredients:

1 batch of any sweet roll dough, pages 217 to 222
1 tsp. grated lemon or orange rind (optional)

¼ c. flour, the same kind as used in the dough recipe
⅓ c. date sugar or granular Fruit Source™
1 tsp. cinnamon
1 to 2 tbsp. oil (use larger amount with rice flour)
2 tbsp. finely chopped walnuts or other nuts

Cycle: Dough cycle using the ingredients above the dotted line. Add the lemon or orange rind to the bread machine pan with the salt. When the cycle finishes, spread the dough in a lightly oiled 9″ by 9″ pan. In a bowl, stir together the flour, sweetener, and cinnamon. With a pastry cutter, cut in the oil. Stir in the nuts. Sprinkle the topping over the dough. Allow it to rise in a warm place until double, 30 to 60 minutes, depending on the kind of dough used. Bake at 375°F for 25 to 40 minutes, or until the coffee cake is browned on the top and bottom.

Nutritional Analysis: To the whole batch values for the dough recipe you used, add 515 calories, 7 g. protein, 73 g. carbohydrate, 22 g. fat, 0.5 g. saturated fat, 2 mg. sodium, and 5 g. fiber. Divide by the number of servings to get the per serving values.

Diabetic exchanges per whole batch: To the whole batch values for the dough recipe used add 1 starch/bread + 5 fat + 3½ fruit. Divide by the number of servings to get the exchanges per serving.

Monkey Bread

Ingredients:

1 batch of any sweet roll dough, pages 217 to 222
Cooking oil spray
⅓ c.   granular Fruit Source™ OR ½ c. date sugar
 2 tsp. cinnamon

Cycle: Dough cycle, using the dough ingredients only. When the cycle finishes, knead the dough briefly on a lightly floured board. Oil a 10″ tube pan or a 2 to 3-qt. round casserole dish. Divide the dough into 45 to 50 1″ balls. Spray each lightly with cooking oil spray and roll it in a mixture of the sweetener and cinnamon. Place the balls in the prepared pan. Sprinkle any remaining cinnamon-sweetener mixture over the top of the balls. Let the bread rise in a warm place until double, about 35 to 50 minutes. Bake at 375°F for 35 to 45 minutes, or until brown. Remove from the pan immediately.

Nutritional analysis: To the whole batch values for the dough you use, add 256 calories, 63 g. carbohydrate, and 32 mg. sodium.

Diabetic exchanges per serving: To the whole batch values for the dough recipe you used, add 4 fruit exchanges. Divide by the total number of servings to get the exchanges per serving.

Fruit Kuchen

Ingredients:

1 batch of any sweet roll dough, pages 217 to 221
4 to 5 cups fresh or frozen blueberries or
    peeled, sliced apples or peaches
½ c. flour, the same kind as used in the dough recipe
½ c. quick cooking oats, uncooked
½ c. date sugar
 3 tsp. cinnamon
 2 tbsp. oil

Cycle: Dough cycle, using the dough recipe ingredients only.
When the cycle finishes, spread the dough in a lightly oiled 9"
by 13" pan. Arrange the fruit evenly over the dough. In a bowl,
stir together the flour, oats, date sugar, and cinnamon. Sprinkle
the mixture with the oil and mix it in with your fingers.
Sprinkle the oat topping over the fruit. Allow the kuchen to rise
in a warm place until double, 30 to 60 minutes, depending on
the kind of dough used. Bake at 350°F for 40 to 50 minutes, or
until browned on the top and bottom.

Nutritional Analysis: To the whole batch values for the dough recipe you used, add
1218 calories, 18 g. protein, 225 g. carbohydrate, 31 g. fat, 37 mg. sodium, and
28 g fiber. Divide by the number of servings to get the per serving values.

Diabetic exchanges per whole batch: To the whole batch values for the dough recipe
used add 5 starch/bread + 11 fruit + 4 fat. Divide by the number of servings to get
the exchanges per serving.

Freeform Apple Pie

Dough ingredients (1½ or 1 lb. machine):

½ c. + 1 tbsp.	water
2 tbsp.	apple juice concentrate, thawed
1 tbsp.	oil
½ tsp.	salt
2 c.	bread flour
1⅛ tsp.	active dry yeast

Filling ingredients:

5 to 6 c.	peeled, sliced apples
1 tsp.	cinnamon
½ c.	date sugar
⅛ c.	tapioca flour or cornstarch

Cycle: Dough cycle, using the dough ingredients. When the cycle is finished, roll the dough out on a floured surface to a 16" circle. Transfer the dough to an oiled baking sheet. Mix the filling ingredients and put them in the center of the dough. Bring the edges of the dough up around the fruit to form a 10" pie, leaving a 5" circle of fruit exposed in the middle. Pleat the dough on the top of the pie and pinch the pleats together. Allow to rise in a warm place for 25 to 30 minutes. Cover the exposed fruit with a small circle of aluminum foil. Bake at 350°F for 40 to 55 minutes, or until brown on the top and bottom.

Nutritional Analysis: (% Daily Value based on a 2000 calorie diet)

	Per Pie	Per serving	%D.V.
Calories:	1847	231	12%
Protein (g):	30	4	-
Carbohydrate (g):	394	49	16%
Total fat (g):	18	2.3	3%
Saturated (g):	0	0	0
Cholesterol (mg):	0	0	0
Sodium (mg):	772	97	4%
Fiber (g):	5.6	0.7	2%

Serving size: ⅛ pie; Servings per batch: 8

Diabetic exchanges per serving: 1½ starch/bread + 2 fruit

Wheat-free Freeform Apple Pie

Dough ingredients (1½ or 1 lb. machine):

½ c.	water
2 tbsp.	apple juice concentrate, thawed
1 tbsp.	oil
⅜ tsp.	salt
2 c.	white spelt flour
1¼ tsp.	active dry yeast

Filling ingredients:

5 to 6 c.	peeled, sliced apples
1 tsp.	cinnamon
½ c.	date sugar
⅛ c.	tapioca flour or cornstarch

Cycle: Dough cycle, using the dough ingredients. When the cycle is finished, roll the dough out on a floured surface to a 16" circle. Transfer the dough to an oiled baking sheet. Mix the filling ingredients and put them in the center of the dough. Bring the edges of the dough up around the fruit to form a 10" pie, leaving a 5" circle of fruit exposed in the middle. Pleat the dough on the top of the pie and pinch the pleats together. Allow to rise in a warm place for 25 to 30 minutes. Cover the exposed fruit with a small circle of aluminum foil. Bake at 350°F for 40 to 55 minutes, or until brown on the top and bottom.

Nutritional Analysis: (% Daily Value based on a 2000 calorie diet)

	Per Pie	Per serving	%D.V.
Calories:	1877	234	12%
Protein (g):	36	4.5	-
Carbohydrate (g):	398	50	16%
Total fat (g):	20	2.5	4%
Saturated (g):	0	0	0
Cholesterol (mg):	0	0	0
Sodium (mg):	772	97	4%
Fiber (g):	4	0.5	2%

Serving size: ⅛ pie; Servings per batch: 8
Diabetic exchanges per serving: 1½ starch/bread + 2 fruit

Open Faced Pie

Dough ingredients (1½ lb. or 1 lb. machine):

⅜ c.   water
1 tbsp. + 1 tsp. apple juice concentrate, thawed
2 tsp.   oil
¼ tsp. salt
1¼ c.   bread flour
¾ tsp. active dry yeast

Cycle: Dough cycle. When the cycle is finished, carefully remove the dough from the machine without deflating it too much. Do not knead it. Roll it out on a lightly floured surface to a 12″ to 13″ circle. Transfer it to an oiled 9″ to 10″ pie plate. Trim the edges and fill with one of the fillings on the following pages. If desired, reroll the scraps of dough and cut into wedges or into small shapes with cookie cutters. Lay them on top of the filling. Allow the pie to raise in a warm place for 25 to 30 minutes. Bake in a preheated 350°F oven for 40 to 50 minutes, covering with foil after the first 25 minutes.

Nutritional Analysis: (% Daily Value based on a 2000 calorie diet. These values are for the crust only and must be added to the values for the filling in the recipes below.)

	Per Pie	Per serving	%D.V.
Calories:	624	78	4%
Protein (g):	17	2.1	-
Carbohydrate (g):	112	14	5%
Total fat (g):	10	1.3	2%
Saturated (g):	0	0	0
Cholesterol (mg):	0	0	0
Sodium (mg):	512	64	3%
Fiber (g):	0.4	0.05	<1%

Serving size: ⅛ pie
Servings per pie: 8

Diabetic exchanges per serving: 1 starch/bread

Wheat-free Open Faced Pie

Dough ingredients (1½ lb. or 1 lb. machine):

⅓ c.   water
1 tbsp. + 1 tsp. apple juice concentrate, thawed
2 tsp. oil
¼ tsp. salt
1⅓ c.   white spelt flour
⅞ tsp. active dry yeast

Cycle: Dough cycle. When the cycle is finished, carefully remove the dough from the machine without deflating it too much. Do not knead it. Roll it out on a lightly floured surface to a 12″ to 13″ circle. Transfer it to an oiled 9″ to 10″ pie plate. Trim the edges and fill with one of the fillings on the following pages. If desired, reroll the scraps of dough and cut into wedges or into small shapes with cookie cutters. Lay them on top of the filling. Allow the pie to raise in a warm place for 25 to 30 minutes. Bake in a preheated 350°F oven for 40 to 50 minutes, covering with foil after the first 25 minutes.

Nutritional Analysis: (% Daily Value based on a 2000 calorie diet. These values are for the crust only and must be added to the values for the filling in the recipes below.)

	Per Pie	Per serving	%D.V.
Calories:	678	85	4%
Protein (g):	22	2.8	-
Carbohydrate (g):	122	15	5%
Total fat (g):	11	1.4	2%
Saturated (g):	0	0	0
Cholesterol (mg):	0	0	0
Sodium (mg):	511	64	3%
Fiber (g):	2	0.3	1%

Serving size: ⅛ pie
Servings per pie: 8

Diabetic exchanges per serving: 1 starch/bread

Pumpkin Open Faced Pie Filling

Filling ingredients:

1 c.   water
1 envelope of unflavored gelatin
    OR 1 tbsp. coarse agar flakes OR 1½ tsp. fine agar flakes
1 16-oz. can pumpkin
1 c.   date sugar
1 tsp.   cinnamon
1 tsp.   nutmeg
¼ tsp.   ground cloves
¼ tsp.   allspice
¼ tsp.   ginger

Prepare the filling while the dough cycle for the pie crust is running. Put the water in a saucepan and sprinkle the gelatin or agar over the surface. Bring it to a boil and simmer until the gelatin or agar dissolves. Stir in the rest of the ingredients thoroughly. Put it into the pie crust prepared as on p. 210 or 211. Allow the pie to rise in a warm place for 25 to 30 minutes. Bake in a preheated 350°F oven for 40 to 50 minutes, covering with foil after the first 25 minutes. Chill thoroughly before serving.

Nutritional Analysis: (% Daily Value based on a 2000 calorie diet. These values are for the filling only and must be added to the values for the crust used.)

	Per Pie	Per serving	%D.V.
Calories:	749	94	5%
Protein (g):	9	1.1	-
Carbohydrate (g):	178	22	7%
Total fat (g):	0	0	0
Saturated (g):	0	0	0
Cholesterol (mg):	0	0	0
Sodium (mg):	45	6	<1%
Fiber (g):	15	1.9	6%

Serving size: ⅛ pie
Servings per pie: 8

Diabetic exchanges per serving: 1¼ fruit + 1 vegetable

Blueberry Open Faced Pie Filling

Filling ingredients:

¾ c. apple juice concentrate, thawed
4 tbsp. quick cooking tapioca granules
24 oz. frozen unsweetened or fresh blueberries

Prepare the filling while the dough cycle for the crust is running. Combine the apple juice and tapioca in a saucepan and allow them to stand for 5 minutes. Stir in the fruit. Bring the mixture to a boil and simmer for 5 minutes. Allow it to cool for at least 30 minutes. Then put it into the pie crust prepared as on p. 210 or 211. Allow the pie to rise in a warm place for 25 to 30 minutes. Bake in a preheated 350°F oven for 40 to 50 minutes, covering with foil after the first 25 minutes.

Nutritional Analysis: (% Daily Value based on a 2000 calorie diet. These values are for the filling only and must be added to the values for the crust used.)

	Per Pie	Per serving	%D.V.
Calories:	831	104	5%
Protein (g):	3	0.4	-
Carbohydrate (g):	205	26	9%
Total fat (g):	0	0	0
Saturated (g):	0	0	0
Cholesterol (mg):	0	0	0
Sodium (mg):	55	7	<1%
Fiber (g):	33	4	14%

Serving size: ⅛ pie
Servings per pie: 8

Diabetic exchanges per serving: 1¾ fruit

Apple Open Faced Pie Filling

Filling ingredients:

¾ c. apple juice concentrate, thawed
2 to 3 tbsp. quick cooking tapioca granules
5 to 6 cups peeled and sliced apples (about 6-7 apples)
1 tsp. cinnamon

Prepare the filling while the dough cycle for the crust is running. Combine the apple juice and tapioca in a saucepan and allow them to stand for 5 minutes. Stir in the fruit. Bring the mixture to a boil and simmer for 10 to 15 minutes, or until the apples soften slightly. Allow the filling to cool for at least 30 minutes. Then put it into the pie crust prepared as on p. 210 or 211. Allow the pie to rise in a warm place for 25 to 30 minutes. Bake in a preheated 350°F oven for 40 to 50 minutes, covering with foil after the first 25 minutes.

Nutritional Analysis: (% Daily Value based on a 2000 calorie diet. These values are for the filling only and must be added to the values for the crust used.)

	Per Pie	Per serving	%D.V.
Calories:	878	110	6%
Protein (g):	2	0.3	-
Carbohydrate (g):	218	27	9%
Total fat (g):	3	0.4	<1%
Saturated (g):	0	0	0
Cholesterol (mg):	0	0	0
Sodium (mg):	56	7	<1%
Fiber (g):	5	0.6	2%

Serving size: ⅛ pie
Servings per pie: 8

Diabetic exchanges per serving: 2 fruit

Cherry Open Faced Pie Filling

Filling ingredients:

1½ c. apple juice concentrate, thawed
4 tbsp. quick cooking tapioca granules
2 16-oz. cans unsweetened
    (water-pack) tart pie cherries, drained

Prepare the filling while the dough cycle for the crust is running. Boil the apple juice down to ¾ c. volume and allow it to cool slightly. Add the tapioca to the saucepan and allow it to stand for 5 minutes. Stir in the fruit. Bring the mixture to a boil and simmer for 5 minutes. Allow it to cool for at least 30 minutes. Then put it into the pie crust prepared as on p. 210 or 211. Allow the pie to rise in a warm place for 25 to 30 minutes. Bake in a preheated 350°F oven for 40 to 50 minutes, covering with foil after the first 25 minutes.

Nutritional Analysis: (% Daily Value based on a 2000 calorie diet. These values are for the filling only and must be added to the values for the crust used.)

	Per Pie	Per serving	%D.V.
Calories:	1114	139	7%
Protein (g):	6	0.8	-
Carbohydrate (g):	272	35	12%
Total fat (g):	1	0.1	<1%
Saturated (g):	0	0	0
Cholesterol (mg):	0	0	0
Sodium (mg):	26	3	<1%
Fiber (g):	7	0.9	3%

Serving size: ⅛ pie
Servings per pie: 8

Diabetic exchanges per serving: 2¼ fruit

Peach Open Faced Pie Filling

Filling ingredients:

¾ c. apple juice concentrate, thawed
4 tbsp. quick cooking tapioca granules
5 c. peeled, pitted, and sliced fresh peaches OR 5 c. drained
     canned water-pack peaches OR 24 oz. frozen unsweetened
     peaches

Prepare the filling while the dough cycle for the crust is running. Combine the apple juice and tapioca in a saucepan and allow them to stand for 5 minutes. Stir in the fruit. Bring the mixture to a boil and simmer for 5 minutes. Allow it to cool for at least 30 minutes. Then put it into the pie crust prepared as on p. 210 or 211. Allow the pie to rise in a warm place for 25 to 30 minutes. Bake in a preheated 350°F oven for 40 to 50 minutes, covering with foil after the first 25 minutes.

Nutritional Analysis: (% Daily Value based on a 2000 calorie diet. These values are for the filling only and must be added to the values for the crust used.)

	Per Pie	Per serving	%D.V.
Calories:	897	112	6%
Protein (g):	6	0.8	-
Carbohydrate (g):	218	27	9%
Total fat (g):	0	0	0
Saturated (g):	0	0	0
Cholesterol (mg):	0	0	0
Sodium (mg):	56	7	<1%
Fiber (g):	20	2.5	8%

Serving size: ⅛ pie
Servings per pie: 8

Diabetic exchanges per serving: 2 fruit

Sweet Rolls and Doughnuts

Sweet Roll Dough

Ingredients:	1½ lb. or 1 lb. machine	
Water	⅞	c.
Fruit Sweet™ or honey	⅓	c.
Oil	1½	tbsp.
Liquid lecithin (or may use additional oil)	1	tbsp.
Salt	¾	tsp.
Bread flour	3⅛	c.
Active dry yeast	1¾	tsp.

Cycle: Dough cycle

Nutritional Analysis: (These values are for the dough only. Add the values for additional ingredients in the following recipes and divide by the number of servings to get the per serving values.)

	Per batch
Calories:	1726
Protein (g):	43
Carbohydrate (g):	298
Total fat (g):	36
Saturated (g):	0
Cholesterol (mg):	0
Sodium (mg):	1514
Fiber (g):	6

Diabetic exchanges per whole batch: 22 starch/bread

White Spelt Sweet Roll Dough

Ingredients: **1½ lb. or 1 lb. machine**

Water	⅔ c.
Fruit Sweet™ or honey	⅓ c.
Oil	1 tbsp.
Liquid lecithin (or may use additional oil)	1 tbsp.
Salt	¾ tsp.
White spelt flour	3¼ c.
Active dry yeast	1¾ tsp.

Cycle: Dough cycle

Nutritional Analysis: (These values are for the dough only. Add the values for additional ingredients in the following recipes and divide by the number of servings to get the per serving values.)

	Per batch
Calories:	1765
Protein (g):	54
Carbohydrate (g):	315
Total fat (g):	34
Saturated (g):	0
Cholesterol (mg):	0
Sodium (mg):	1514
Fiber (g):	19

Diabetic exchanges per whole batch: 22 starch/bread

Whole Wheat Sweet Roll Dough

Ingredients:

	1½ lb. or 1 lb. machine
Water	1 c.
Fruit Sweet™ or honey	⅓ c.
Oil	1 tbsp.
Liquid lecithin (or may use additional oil)	1 tbsp.
Salt	½ tsp.
Whole wheat flour	3 c.
Active dry yeast	2¼ tsp.

Cycle: Dough cycle

Nutritional Analysis: (These values are for the dough only. Add the values for additional ingredients in the following recipes and divide by the number of servings to get the per serving values.)

	Per batch
Calories:	1860
Protein (g):	56
Carbohydrate (g):	326
Total fat (g):	37
Saturated (g):	0
Cholesterol (mg):	0
Sodium (mg):	1021
Fiber (g):	14

Diabetic exchanges per whole batch: 23 starch/bread

Whole Spelt Sweet Roll Dough

Ingredients:	1½ lb. or 1 lb. machine
Water	1 c.
Fruit Sweet™ or honey	⅓ c.
Oil	1 tbsp.
Liquid lecithin (or may use additional oil)	1 tbsp.
Salt	½ tsp.
Whole spelt flour	3¾ c.
Active dry yeast	2¼ tsp.

Cycle: Dough cycle

Nutritional Analysis: (These values are for the dough only. Add the values for additional ingredients in the following recipes and divide by the number of servings to get the per serving values.)

	Per batch
Calories:	2032
Protein (g):	63
Carbohydrate (g):	358
Total fat (g):	38
Saturated (g):	0
Cholesterol (mg):	0
Sodium (mg):	1017
Fiber (g):	35

Diabetic exchanges per whole batch: 25 starch/bread

Kamut Sweet Roll Dough

Ingredients:	**1½ lb. or 1 lb. machine**
Water	1⅛ c.
Fruit Sweet™ or honey	⅜ c.
Oil	1 tbsp.
Liquid lecithin (or may use additional oil)	1 tbsp.
Salt	½ tsp.
Kamut flour	3¼ c.
Active dry yeast	2¼ tsp.

Cycle: Dough cycle

Nutritional Analysis: (These values are for the dough only. Add the values for additional ingredients in the following recipes and divide by the number of servings to get the per serving values.)

	Per batch
Calories:	2414
Protein (g):	65
Carbohydrate (g):	471
Total fat (g):	31
Saturated (g):	0
Cholesterol (mg):	0
Sodium (mg):	1512
Fiber (g):	77

Diabetic exchanges per whole batch: 30 starch/bread

Gluten-free Sweet Roll Dough

Ingredients:	1½ lb. or 1 lb. machine
Water	½ c.
Fruit Sweet™ or honey	¼ c.
Oil	2 tbsp.
Eggs OR egg substitute	3 eggs OR ¾ c.
Salt	1 tsp.
Vitamin C crystals	⅛ tsp.
Guar gum	4 tsp.
Brown rice flour	2 c.
Potato flour	⅓ c.
Tapioca flour	⅓ c.
Active dry yeast	2¼ tsp.

Cycle: Dough cycle. This dough can be used in Streusel Coffee Cake, p.205, Cinnamon Rolls, p.226, or Monkey Bread, p.206.

Nutritional Analysis: (These values are for the dough only. Add the values for additional ingredients in the following recipes and divide by the number of servings to get the per serving values.)

	Per batch
Calories (with eggs):	1900
(with egg substitute):	1892
Protein (g):	54
Carbohydrate (g):	328
Total fat (g) (eggs):	52
(with egg substitute):	61
Saturated (g) (eggs):	5
(egg substitute):	0
Cholesterol (mg) (eggs):	1029
(with egg substitute):	0
Sodium (mg) (eggs):	2269
(with egg substitute):	2344
Fiber (g):	21

Diabetic exchanges per whole batch: 24 starch/bread

Sweet Roll Glaze

Ingredients:

½ c. powdered sugar
2 tsp. water

Mix together thoroughly and drizzle on sweet bread or rolls.

Nutritional Analysis: To the whole batch values for the rolls or bread you use this glaze on add 240 calories and 60 g. carbohydrate.

Diabetic exchanges: Not recommended for diabetics since this is almost pure sugar.

Lemon Sweet Roll Glaze

Ingredients:

½ c. powdered sugar
1 tbsp. lemon juice

Mix together thoroughly and drizzle on sweet bread or rolls.

Nutritional Analysis: To the whole batch values for the rolls or bread you use this glaze on add 244 calories and 61 g. carbohydrate.

Diabetic exchanges: Not recommended for diabetics since this is almost pure sugar.

Orange Sweet Roll Glaze

Ingredients:

½ c. powdered sugar
5 tsp. orange juice concentrate, thawed

Mix together thoroughly and drizzle on sweet bread or rolls.

Nutritional Analysis: To the whole batch values for the rolls or bread you use this glaze on add 288 calories, 1 g. protein, and 71 g. carbohydrate.

Diabetic exchanges: Not recommended for diabetics since this is almost pure sugar.

Pineapple Sweet Roll Glaze

Ingredients:

½ c. powdered sugar
2 tbsp. pineapple juice concentrate, thawed

Mix together thoroughly and drizzle on sweet bread or rolls.

Nutritional Analysis: To the whole batch values for the rolls or bread you use this glaze on add 308 calories, 1 g. protein, and 76 g. carbohydrate.

Diabetic exchanges: Not recommended for diabetics since this is almost pure sugar.

Hot Cross Buns

Ingredients:

1 batch of any sweet roll dough, pages 217 to 221
½ c. currants or dried blueberries
1 slightly beaten egg white or "Bread or Bun Wash," p. 129
Any sweet roll glaze, pages 223 to 224, optional

Cycle: Dough cycle, using the dough ingredients only. Add the currants or raisins to the machine 5 to 10 minutes before the end of the last kneading time. At the end of the cycle, remove the dough from the machine and knead it a few times on a lightly oiled board. Roll it to ½" thickness with a lightly oiled rolling pin. Cut rounds of dough with a 2½" biscuit cutter or glass. Place them on a baking sheet that has been sprayed with cooking oil spray or lightly oiled and allow them to rise in a warm place until double, about 40 minutes. Snip a shallow cross in the top of each bun with a very sharp scissors, knife, or lame. Brush the tops of the rolls with the egg white or wash. Bake at 375°F for 15 minutes, or until lightly browned. If desired, use sweet roll glaze to pipe a cross into the cross cut on the top of each roll. Makes about 12 buns.

Nutritional Analysis: To the whole batch values for the dough recipe used add 220 calories, 3 g. protein, 52 g. carbohydrate, 5 mg. sodium, and 1 g. fiber. Divide the total by the number of servings made to get the per serving values.

Diabetic exchanges per batch: To the whole batch values for the dough used add 4 fruit exchanges. Divide by the number of servings made to get the number of exchanges per serving.

Cinnamon Rolls

Ingredients:
1 batch of any sweet roll dough, pages 217 to 222
Cooking oil spray OR 2 tsp. oil
½ c. date sugar OR granular fruit source
   (if you must, substitute ¼ c. sugar)
2 tsp. cinnamon
½ c. raisins
Any sweet roll glaze, pages 223 to 224 (optional)

Cycle: Dough cycle with the sweet roll dough ingredients. When the cycle is finished, remove the dough from the machine and use a lightly oiled rolling pin to roll it out to a 12″ by 15″ or longer rectangle on a lightly oiled board. Spray the rectangle with cooking oil spray or brush it with oil. Sprinkle it with the sweetener, cinnamon, and raisins. Starting at the long side, roll the dough up jelly roll fashion. Cut the roll into 12 to 15 slices and put them cut side down in an oiled 13″ by 9″ pan. (Or for individual cinnamon rolls, cut the dough into 15 slices and put each slice cut side down into an oiled muffin cup.) Allow them to rise in a warm place until double, about 35 to 50 minutes. Bake at 375°F for 20 to 30 minutes. Drizzle with any sweet roll glaze if desired.

To make cinnamon rolls with gluten-free dough, when you remove the dough from the machine, pat it out into a 6″ by 12″ rectangle on a very well oiled board. Spray or brush it with oil. Sprinkle it with ¼ c. date sugar or fruit source, 1½ tsp. cinnamon, and ¼ c. raisins. Roll it up carefully starting at the long edge and cut it into 9 slices. Put them in an oiled 8″ or 9″ square baking pan and allow to rise until double, about 30 minutes. Bake as above. The nutritional values to add to the values for the dough are half of those given below.

Nutritional Analysis: To the whole batch values for the dough recipe used add 611 calories, 2 g. protein, 150 g. carbohydrate, 57 mg. sodium, and 6 g. fiber. Divide the total by the number of servings made to get the per serving values.

Diabetic exchanges per batch: 10 fruit. Add to the exchanges per batch for the dough used and divide by the number of servings made to get the number of exchanges per serving.

Heart Healthy Doughnuts

Ingredients:

1 batch of any sweet roll dough, pages 217 to 221
Cooking oil spray
1 batch of any doughnut topping or frosting,
    pages 228 to 230 (optional)

Cycle: Dough cycle. When the cycle is finished, roll the dough out to about ½" thickness on a lightly oiled board with an oiled rolling pin. Cut into doughnuts with a floured doughnut cutter. Lightly oil a baking sheet or spray it with cooking oil spray. Transfer the doughnuts to the sheet with a spatula and spray them lightly with cooking oil spray. Let them rise in a warm place until double, about 30 to 40 minutes. Bake at 375°F for 10 to 15 minutes, or until the doughnuts are just beginning to brown. Spray both the top and bottom of each doughnut lightly with cooking oil spray and immediately shake them in one of the toppings below. Or, if you wish to frost them, allow them to cool before frosting them with one of the frostings below.

Nutritional Analysis: Essentially the same as for the dough used. Divide the whole batch values for the dough used by the number of doughnuts made to get the values for each doughnut.

Diabetic exchanges per doughnut: Divide the number of exchanges for a whole batch of the dough used by the number of doughnuts made to get the exchanges per serving.

Cinnamon "Sugar" Doughnut Topping

Ingredients:
¼ c. granular Fruit Source™ (or if you must, substitute sugar)
1 tsp cinnamon

Mix the sweetener and cinnamon in a plastic bag. After baking the doughnuts, spray each one with cooking oil spray and shake them one at a time in the bag with the cinnamon mixture while still warm.

Nutritional Analysis: To the whole batch values for the dough recipe used add 192 calories, 48 g. carbohydrate, and 24 mg. sodium. Divide the total by the number of doughnuts made to get the per doughnut values.

Diabetic exchanges per batch: To the whole batch values for the dough used add 3 fruit exchanges. Divide by the number of doughnuts made to get the number of exchanges per doughnut.

Powdered "Sugar" Doughnut Topping

Ingredients:
¼ c. banana powder* OR powdered sugar

Put the banana powder or powdered sugar in a plastic bag. After baking the doughnuts, spray each one with cooking oil spray and shake them one at a time in the bag with the powder while still warm.

*Banana powder, which is dehydrated ground bananas, can be purchased from The King Arthur Flour Baker's Catalogue. (See "Sources," p. 235.)

Nutritional Analysis: For the banana powder, to the whole batch values for the dough recipe used add 220 calories, 2 g. protein, 53 g. carbohydrate, and 2 mg. sodium. For the powdered sugar, to the whole batch values for the dough recipe used add 120 calories and 30 g. carbohydrate. Divide the total by the number of doughnuts made to get the per doughnut values.

Diabetic exchanges per batch: 4 fruit for the banana powder. Add to the exchanges per batch for the dough used and divide by the number of doughnuts made to get the number of exchanges per doughnut.

White Doughnut Frosting

Ingredients:
¾ c. powdered sugar
2½ to 3½ tsp. water

Mix the sugar with enough water to make a thick frosting. Spread on the doughnuts and sprinkle with nuts or coconut if desired.

Nutritional Analysis: To the whole batch values for the dough recipe used add 360 calories and 90 g. carbohydrate. Divide the total by the number of doughnuts made to get the per doughnut values.

Diabetic exchanges per batch: Not recommended for diabetics since this is almost pure sugar.

Chocolate Doughnut Frosting

Ingredients:
½ c. powdered sugar
2 tbsp. cocoa
2½ to 3½ tsp. water

Mix the sugar and cocoa with enough water to make a thick frosting. Spread on the doughnuts and sprinkle with nuts or coconut if desired.

Nutritional Analysis: To the whole batch values for the dough recipe used add 274 calories, 2 g. protein, 62 g. carbohydrate, 2 g. fat, and 1 mg. sodium. Divide the total by the number of doughnuts made to get the per doughnut values.

Diabetic exchanges per batch: Not recommended for diabetics since this is almost pure sugar.

Orange Rolls

Ingredients:
1 batch of any sweet roll dough, pages 217 to 221
3 tsp. oil
½ c. granular Fruit Source™ (may substitute sugar if you must)
4 tsp. grated orange peel, divided
"Orange Glaze," p. 224 (optional)

Cycle: Dough cycle, adding 2 tsp. grated orange peel to the machine with the salt. When the cycle is finished, remove the dough from the machine and divide it in half. Roll each half out to a 12″ by 7″ rectangle on a lightly oiled board. Brush each half with 1½ tsp. oil. Sprinkle each half with ¼ c. granular Fruit Source™ and 1 tsp. grated orange peel. Roll up jelly roll fashion starting with the long side. Cut each roll into 12 slices and place them cut side down on an oiled or non-stick baking sheet. Let rise until double, about 30 to 35 minutes. Bake at 375°F for 12 to 18 minutes. Cool and drizzle with "Orange Glaze," if desired.

Nutritional Analysis: To the whole batch values for the dough recipe used add 516 calories, 96 g. carbohydrate, 13 g. fat, and 48 mg. sodium. Divide the total by 24 to get the per serving values.

Diabetic exchanges per batch: To the exchanges per batch for the dough used add 3 fruit + 1½ fat exchanges. Divide 24 to get the number of exchanges per serving.

Lemon Rolls

Make the same as "Orange Rolls," above, except substitute lemon peel for the orange peel and drizzle with "Lemon Glaze," p. 223, if desired.

Nutritional Analysis: Same as for "Orange Rolls," above

Diabetic Exchanges: Same as for "Orange Rolls," above

Cinnamon Crisps

Ingredients:
1 batch of any sweet roll dough, pages 217 to 221
2 tsp. oil
⅓ c. + ¼ c. granular Fruit Source™
   (may substitute sugar if you must)
2½ tsp. cinnamon, divided
Cooking oil spray
½ c. chopped walnuts or other nuts

Cycle: Dough cycle, using only the sweet roll dough ingredients. When the cycle is finished, remove the dough from the machine and divide it in half. On an oiled board, use a lightly oiled rolling pin to roll each half out to a 12″ square. Brush each half with 1 tsp. oil. Sprinkle each half with about ⅙ c. sweetener and ¾ tsp. cinnamon. Roll the dough up jelly roll fashion. Cut the roll into 12 slices and put them cut side down at least 3″ apart on an oiled baking sheet. Oil your hand and flatten the slices with your fingers to make them about 3″ in diameter. (They may spring back some after you remove your hand.) Allow them to rise in a warm place until double, about 30 minutes. Spray the tops of the rolls lightly with cooking oil spray and cover them with a piece of waxed or parchment paper. Use a rolling pin to flatten them to ⅛″ to ¼″ thickness. Mix together the remaining ¼ c. sweetener, 1 tsp. cinnamon, and nuts. Sprinkle the cinnamon crisps with the mixture. Cover them with the waxed or parchment paper and flatten them to ⅛″ to ¼″ thickness again. Bake at 400°F for 10 to 12 minutes.

Nutritional Analysis: To the whole batch values for the dough recipe used add 887 calories, 13 g. protein, 118 g. carbohydrate, 39 g. fat, 2 g. saturated fat, 58 mg. sodium, and 5 g. fiber. Divide the total by 24 to get the per serving values.

Diabetic exchanges per batch: To the whole batch values for the dough recipe used add 9 fruit + 8 fat exchanges. Divide 24 to get the number of exchanges per serving.

Heart Healthy Danish

Ingredients:
1 batch of any sweet roll dough, pages 217 to 221
2 tsp. oil
⅓ c. + ¼ c. granular Fruit Source™
   (may substitute sugar if you must)
2½ tsp. cinnamon, divided
Cooking oil spray
½ c. chopped walnuts or other nuts
¼ c. all fruit (sugar-free) jam

Cycle: Dough cycle, using only the sweet roll dough ingredients. When the cycle is finished, remove the dough from the machine and divide it in half. On an oiled board, use a lightly oiled rolling pin to roll each half out to a 12″ square. Brush each half with 1 tsp. oil. Sprinkle each half with about ⅙ c. sweetener and ¾ tsp. cinnamon. Roll the dough up jelly roll fashion. Cut the roll into 12 slices and put them cut side down at least 3″ apart on an oiled baking sheet. Oil your hand and flatten the slices with your fingers to make them about 3″ in diameter. (They may spring back some after you remove your hand.) Allow them to rise in a warm place until double, about 30 to 40 minutes. Spray the tops of the rolls lightly with cooking oil spray and cover them with a piece of waxed or parchment paper. Use a rolling pin to flatten them to ¼″ to ⅜″ thickness. Mix together the remaining ¼ c. sweetener, 1 tsp. cinnamon, and nuts. Sprinkle the rolls with the mixture. Cover them with the waxed or parchment paper and flatten them to ¼″ to ⅜″ thickness again. Let them rise until double again, about 30 to 40 minutes. Make an indentation in the center of each roll with your fingertip and fill it with ½ tsp. jam. Bake at 375°F for 8 to 12 minutes. Drizzle with any sweet roll glaze, pages 223 to 224, if desired.

Nutritional Analysis: To the whole batch values for the dough recipe used add 1077 calories, 13 g. protein, 168 g. carbohydrate, 39 g. fat, 2 g. saturated fat, 65 mg. sodium, and 5 g. fiber. Divide the total by 24 to get the per serving values.

Diabetic exchanges per batch: To the whole batch values for the dough recipe used add 12 fruit + 8 fat exchanges. Divide 24 to get the number of exchanges per serving.

References

American Diabetes Association/American Dietetic Association, *Family Cookbook,* Volumes I, II, and III, Prentice-Hall, Inc., Englewood Cliffs, NJ 07632, 1980, 1984, and 1987.

American Heart Association, *American Heart Association Cookbook,* Random House, Inc., New York, NY 10022, 1991.

Crook, William G., M.D., *Detecting Your Hidden Allergies,* Professional Books, 681 Skyline Drive, Jackson, TN 38301, 1988.

Dumke, Nicolette M., *Allergy Cooking With Ease,* Starburst Publishers, P.O. Box 4123, Lancaster, PA 17604, 1992.

Dumke, Nicolette M., *5 Years Without Food: The Food Allergy Survival Guide,* Allergy Adapt, Inc., 1877 Polk Avenue, Lousiville, CO 80027, 1998.

German, Donna Rathmell and Ed Wood, *Worldwide Sourdoughs from Your Bread Machine,* Bristol Publishing Enterprises, Inc., P.O. Box 1737, San Leandro, CA 94577, 1994.

Jones, Marjorie H., *"Mastering Food Allergies"* Newsletter, Mast Enterprises, Inc., 2615 N. Fourth St., #616, Coeur d'Alene, ID 83814.

Lai, Ada., *"The Magic Bread Letter"* Newsletter, The Magic Bread Letter, P.O. Box 337, Moss Beach, CA 94038.

Rehberg, Linda and Lois Conway, *The Bread Machine Magic Book of Helpful Hints,* St. Martin's Press, 175 Fifth Avenue, New York, NY 10010, 1993.

Scala, James, *Eating Right For a Bad Gut,* Penguin Books USA, Inc., 375 Hudson Street, New York, NY 10014, 1990.

Starke, Rodman D., M.D. and Mary Winston, Ed.D., R.D., *American Heart Association Low-Salt Cookbook,* Random House, Inc., New York, NY 10022, 1990.

Sources of Special Foods and Products

BAKING POWDER, CORN-FREE:

Featherweight Baking Powder
Estee Corporation
169 Lackawanna Avenue
Parsippany, New Jersey 07054
(800) 343-7833

BREAD BOXES, BREAD KNIVES, ETC.;

The King Arthur Flour Baker's Catalogue
P.O. Box 876
Norwich, Vermont 05055
(800) 827-6836

BREAD MACHINES

(Mail order sources):

At the time of this writing, both programmable machines discussed in this book have been discontinued. However, Regal makes machines with a "bake only" cycle that will achieve the same results. See page 248 for how to use this type of machine.

Regal models (including the K-6725) are available in department stores, usually for under $150. If you cannot find a machine locally, they can be mail-ordered from:

Regal Ware, Inc.
  Attention: Carol Heller, Manager Consumer Service
1675 Reigle Drive
Kewaskum, Wisconsin 53040
(414) 626-8502

Zojirushi BBCC-S15: At the time of this writing, this machine may be ordered from Allergy Resources for $320 plus shipping and sales tax where applicable.

Allergy Resources, Inc.
557 Burbank Street, Suite K
Broomfield, Colorado 80020
(800) USE-FLAX

FLOUR:

ALMOST ALL TYPES OF FLOUR, INCLUDING UNBLEACHED, UNBROMATED BREAD FLOUR, WHITE RYE, WHITE WHEAT, ETC.:

> The King Arthur Flour Baker's Catalogue
> P.O. Box 876
> Norwich, Vermont 05055
> (800) 827-6836

ALMOST ALL TYPES OF FLOUR, INCLUDING BUCKWHEAT, RYE, WHITE RICE, BROWN RICE, KAMUT, ETC.

> Arrowhead Mills, Inc.
> 110 South Lawton
> Hereford, Texas 79045
> (806) 364-0730

AMARANTH FLOUR:

> Allergy Resources, Inc. (See address on p. 235.)

> Nu-World Amaranth, Inc.
> P.O. Box 2202
> Naperville, Illinois 60540
> (708) 369-6819

KAMUT FLOUR:

> Arrowhead Mills, Inc.
> 110 South Lawton
> Hereford, Texas 79045
> (806) 364-0730

> Montana Flour & Grains
> Ferry Route, P.O. Box 808
> Big Sandy, Montana 59520
> (406) 378-3105 or (406) 622-5503

POTATO FLOUR, WHITE RICE FLOUR, AND MANY OTHER TYPES OF FLOUR:

> Bob's Red Mill
> Natural Foods Inc.
> 5209 S.E. International Way
> Milwaukie, OR 97222
> (503) 654-3215

QUINOA FLOUR:

>Allergy Resources, Inc. (See address on p. 235.)
>
>The Quinoa Corporation
>P.O. Box 1039
>Torrance, California 90505
>(310) 530-8666

SPELT FLOUR (PURITY FOODS WHOLE AND WHITE SPELT):

>Allergy Resources, Inc. (See address on p. 235.)
>
>Purity Foods, Inc.
>2871 W. Jolly Road
>Okemos, Michigan 48864
>(517) 351-0231

FRUIT SOURCE™:

>Fruit Source
>1803 Mission Street, Suite 404
>Santa Cruz, California 95060
>(408) 457-1136

FRUIT SWEET™:

>The King Arthur Flour Baker's Catalogue (See address
>on page 235.)
>
>Wax Orchards
>22744 Wax Orchards Road., S.W.
>Vashon Island, Washington 98070
>(800) 634-6132

GUAR GUM:

>Allergy Resources, Inc. (See address on p. 235.)
>
>NOW Natural Foods
>550 W. Mitchell
>Glendale Heights, Illinois 60139
>(800) 283-3500

MISCELLANEOUS BREAD INGREDIENTS

(Banana powder, Heidelberg rye sour, etc.)

> The King Arthur Flour Baker's Catalogue
> (See address on page 235.)

SOURDOUGH CULTURES:

> Sourdoughs International, Inc.
> P.O. Box 993
> Cascade, ID 83611

UNBUFFERED VITAMIN C CRYSTALS, ALLERGY SUPPLIES:

> An Ounce of Prevention
> 8200 E. Phillips Place
> Englewood, CO 80112
> (303) 770-8808

XANTHUM GUM:

> Bob's Red Mill (See address on p. 236.)

YEAST:

> Red Star Yeast
> Universal Foods Corporation
> Consumer Service Center
> 433 E. Michigan
> Milwaukee, Wisconsin 53202
> (414) 271-6755

Index of Gluten-free & Wheat-free Recipes by Grain Used

For gluten-free recipes that are acceptable on celiac diets, see the "Rice" section on p. 240. All of the recipes in this index are wheat-free.

General Index

Recipes appear in italics; informational sections appear in standard type.

I

J

K

L

M

N

O

Bread Machine Updates

Like car manufacturers, bread machine manufacturers change their products often. Since the first printing of this book, both the Welbilt ABM-150R and the Zojirushi BBCC-S15 have been discontinued. The newest truly programmable machine on the market is the Breadman Ultimate. However, even though it is programmable, it is not satisfactory for making most allergy breads because it kneads the dough quite violently.

Several companies have introduced new machines with quick bread or cake cycles for non-yeast breads. A few of these machines mix the dough for a very long time before baking. The ideal mixing time for the recipes in this book is 3 to 4 minutes. If your machine mixes longer than 4 minutes, add the oil, but delay adding the other liquid ingredients until about 2 minutes before the end of the mixing time. For example, if it mixes for 6 minutes, rather than adding the liquids 1½ to 2 minutes into the cycle, wait until 4 minutes after you start the machine.

Regal makes several machines that are good for those who need a truly programmable machine because they have dough only and bake only cycles that can be used together to make breads that require a short last rise or to make quick breads. The model I tested was the K-6725, which makes a 1½ to 2 pound loaf of bread. To make a recipe that lists a programmed cycle with this machine, add the ingredients to the pan, put it in the machine, and start the dough cycle. Set your kitchen timer for 40 minutes plus the length of the Rise 2 time listed in the recipe. When it rings, or when the dough appears to have almost doubled in bulk, stop the dough cycle and start the bake cycle. To make quick bread recipes from this book using the Regal machine, DO NOT use the quick bread cycle. Instead, use the dough cycle and proceed as in the mixing directions on p. 144. When the dough is mixed (3 to 4 minutes), stop the dough cycle and start the bake cycle. Because you control when this machine advances from mixing to baking, if you work quickly, you can substitute 1 tsp. baking soda PLUS ¼ tsp. unbuffered vitamin C crystals for the 2½ to 3 tsp. baking powder specified in the recipes.

To make quick breads with the Regal K-6725 or any other machine which has a rectangular rather than a square-bottomed pan, multiply the amounts of all the ingredients in the recipes in this book by 1½ to produce a loaf of normal height.

If you are going to bake yeast breads made with wheat, kamut, or spelt only and have a family which consumes a lot of bread, West Bend's "Baker's Choice" or "Homestyle Plus" machine may be the machine for you. It has a 2-pound horizontally rectangular pan, so you can make very large loaves of both yeast breads and quick breads and bake less frequently. To use this machine with the yeast bread recipes in this book, double the amounts of the ingredients given for a 1 pound loaf. For quick breads, the amounts may also be doubled, adding all of the ingredients to the pan before starting the cycle beginning with the liquid ingredients, then adding the flours and other dry ingredients, and putting the baking powder on the top. This machine also has a front-opening door.

Order Form

ITEM	QUANTITY	PRICE	TOTAL
Easy Breadmaking for Special Diets		$14.95	
Five Years Without Food: The Food Allergy Survival Guide		$19.95	
Allergy Cooking With Ease		$14.95	
The EPD Patient's Cooking and Lifestyle Guide		$6.95	
How to Cope With Food Allergies When You're Short on Time		$2.95 or FREE	

Order any 2 of the first four books above and get *How to Cope with Food Allergies when You're Short on Time* **FREE!**	SUBTOTAL	
	SHIPPING (see table below)	
	Colorado residents add 3.8% sales tax	
	TOTAL	

Ship to:

NAME:

STREET ADDRESS:

CITY, STATE, ZIP

PHONE NUMBER (in case of questions about order):

Please make check payable to:
Allergy Adapt, Inc. and send it and this order to:
Allergy Adapt, Inc., 1877 Polk Ave., Louisville, CO 80027

SHIPPING TABLE

SINGLE TITLE ORDERS:

Easy Breadmaking for Special Diets . . . . .add $3.00

Five Years Without Food: The Food Allergies Survival Guide . . . . .add $4.00

Allergy Cooking With Ease . . . . .add $3.00

The EPD Patient's Cooking and Lifestyle Guide . . . . .add $2.00

How to Cope With Food Allergies When You're Short on Time . . . .add $1.50

MULTIPLE TITLE ORDERS: add $5.00 or the sum of the shipping charges for single titles, whichever is less.

Books to Help You
With Your Special Diet

Easy Breadmaking for Special Diets: 195 recipes for allergy, heart healthy, low fat, low sodium, high or low fiber, diabetic, celiac, and low calorie diets. Includes recipes for breads of all kinds, main dishes, and desserts. Use your bread machine, food processor, or mixer to make the bread YOU need quickly and easily. $14.95

Five Years Without Food: The Food Allergy Survival Guide gives you medical information about the diagnosis of food allergies, health problems that can be caused by food allergies, and your options for treatment. It includes a rotation diet that is free from common food allergens such as wheat, milk, eggs, corn, soy, yeast, beef, legumes, citrus fruits, potatoes, tomatoes, and more. The book contains over 500 recipe variations that are geared to this diet. Instructions are given on how to personalize the standard rotation diet to meet your individual needs and fit your food preferences. Extensive reference sections include a listing of commercially prepared foods for your diet. The producers' addresses and phone numbers are given so you can order these foods directly, or you can get them at your health food store. $19.95

Allergy Cooking With Ease: 250 recipes for wheat-, milk-, egg-, corn-, soy-, and yeast- free diets. Finished in 1991, this is a general allergy cookbook including recipes for a wide variety of baked goods, main dishes including complex casseroles, and desserts including sugar-sweetened desserts for special occasions. $14.95

The EPD Patient's Cooking and Lifestyle Guide: 79 recipes for patients on enzyme potentiated desensitization treatment for their food allergies. Also includes organizational information to help you get ready for your shots. $6.95

How to Cope With Food Allergies When You're Short on Time: Time saving tips and recipes to help you stick to your allergy diet with the least amount of time and effort. $2.95 or FREE

To order these books, see the other side of this page.